POST MORTEM EXAMINATION AND AUTOPSY - CURRENT ISSUES FROM DEATH TO LABORATORY ANALYSIS

Edited by **Kamil Hakan Dogan**

Post Mortem Examination and Autopsy - Current Issues From Death to Laboratory Analysis
http://dx.doi.org/10.5772/intechopen.68970
Edited by Kamil Hakan Dogan

Contributors

Zerrin Erkol, Erdem Hösükler, Hiroshi Kinoshita, Naoko Tanaka, Ayaka Takakura, Padar Zsolt, Petra Zenke, Zsolt Kozma, Abdo Jurjus, Kawthar Braysh, Raymond Zerbe, Rosalyn Jurjus Zein, Jihad Hawi, Doureid Oueidat, Luc Oke, F. Deniz Uzuner, Nilufer Darendeliler, Emine Kaygisiz, Oscar Campuzano, Georgia Sarquella-Brugada, Sergi Cesar, Anna Fernandez-Falgueras, Maria Dolores Zambrano, Anna Iglesias, Josep Brugada, Ramon Brugada, Eric Emile Clua, Dennis Reid, Kamil Hakan Dogan

Published by InTech
Janeza Trdine 9, 51000 Rijeka, Croatia

Publishing Process Manager Marina Dusevic
Technical Editor SPi Global
Cover InTech Design team

First published February, 2018
Printed in Croatia
Legal deposit, Croatia: National and University Library in Zagreb

Additional hard copies can be obtained from orders@intechopen.com

Post Mortem Examination and Autopsy - Current Issues From Death to Laboratory Analysis, Edited by Kamil Hakan Dogan
p. cm.
Print ISBN 978-953-51-3792-4
Online ISBN 978-953-51-3793-1

For EU product safety concerns:
IN TECH d.o.o., Prolaz Marije Krucifikse Kozulić 3, 51000 Rijeka, Croatia,
info@intechopen.com or visit our website at intechopen.com.

Meet the editor

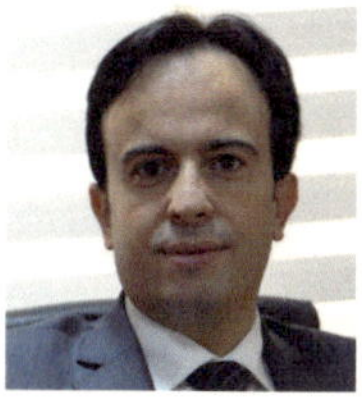

Kamil Hakan Dogan, MD, PhD, is a full professor and chair of the Department of Forensic Medicine, Faculty of Medicine at Selcuk University in Turkey. Dr. Dogan received his MD from Gazi University Faculty of Medicine in 2000. After his extensive researches in Forensic Medicine field, he received his PhD in Biochemistry in 2012. He gives lectures about Forensic Medicine and Medical Ethics to medical students as well as students of dentistry and law faculties. He is a reviewer in several international journals and he has published over 170 articles in refereed journals, chapters in textbooks, and abstracts in scientific meetings. His publications were cited more than 400 times.

Contents

Preface

Post mortem examination remains a benchmark in the study of human disease, and it is a vital tool for teaching anatomy to medical students. But if the death is suspicious, post mortem examination of the body is performed with the intent of determining the cause and manner of the death. Forensic medicine explores the legal aspects of medicine, and medicolegal investigation of death is the most significant and crucial function of it. There is a keen interest among forensic medicine experts and general public about the advancements in forensic medicine. The nature of post mortem examinations is changing, and the understanding of causes of death are evolving with the increase of knowledge, availability, and use of various analyses including genetic testing. Post mortem examination practice is turning into a more multidisciplinary approach for investigations, which are becoming more evidence based.

Death scene investigation, post mortem examination, and autopsy are generally performed for the benefit of the living. A death investigation begins with body examination and evidence collection at the scene and proceeds through history, post mortem examination and autopsy, laboratory tests and determining the cause and manner of death. Forensic pathology is the oldest branch of forensic sciences, and today many branches of forensic sciences play a role in solving criminal death cases.

Although there are numerous publications about forensic medicine and post mortem examination, this book intends to provide some basic information on post mortem examination and current developments in some important and special areas. It is considered that this book will be useful for forensic pathologists, clinicians, attorneys, law enforcement officers, and medical students. I gratefully acknowledge the help and support of the authors from four continents and eight countries of the world who contributed to this book.

Kamil Hakan Dogan
Selcuk University Faculty of Medicine,
Department of Forensic Medicine,
Konya, Turkey

Chapter 1

Introductory Chapter: An Overview of Post-Mortem Examination and Autopsy

Kamil Hakan Dogan and Serafettin Demirci

Additional information is available at the end of the chapter

http://dx.doi.org/10.5772/intechopen.73279

1. Forensic medicine and death investigation

It is obvious that there is an interest in determining the causes of death of its members even in a primitive tribal society. A sudden, unexpected or unwitnessed death must have signaled a potential danger, either by its own members from within the society or by an enemy from the outside [1]. Forensic medicine mainly deals with examination and assessment of individuals who have been—or are suspected to have been—injured or killed by external influence such as trauma or intoxication. In many countries, forensic medicine represents a medical specialty within the legal system, not within the healthcare system [2]. The primary goal of death investigation is establishing the cause and manner of death. The people commonly ask, "The person is dead. Why does it matter?" Yes, the dead cannot benefit, but the value of the death investigation is to benefit the living and future generations. In a culture that values life, it is very important to explain the meaning of death in a public forum ("forensic") [3]. In cases of sudden death, the forensic pathologist determines the cause of death, and his views in criminal cases are crucial to ensuring justice. Data obtained from investigating accidental and suicidal deaths are vital for preventive strategies [4].

2. Who is forensic pathologist?

Forensic pathology is the part of forensic medicine dealing with examination of deceased persons. A common principle is that in the investigation of a possible or suspected criminal death, a forensic pathologist is engaged through a formal request from the police or the prosecutor. The task of the forensic pathologist is then to assist in the investigation as a medical expert. This expert role continues throughout the process, including the court proceedings on request of the court and/or one of the parties [2]. When a physician cannot certify the cause of death in deaths from natural causes and when bodily damage is the major finding, forensic pathologist has to deal mostly with the pathology of accidental (unintentional) and homicidal or suicidal (intentional) trauma. The primary role of forensic pathologist is to determine the cause of death based on a complete autopsy. The forensic medicine expert deals with the examination of the injured person or deceased to determine the cause and nature of the injuries and death in cases involving injuries. In cases of domestic violence, sexual assault, torture, and alleged medical negligence, forensic pathologist's role is very important. Forensic pathologists are like any other forensic scientist in many ways. They identify/classify things and compare them with known examples to confirm or refute hypotheses. The difference is their area of study and examination: the human body. In this sense, they learn what other medical doctors learn: how the body's systems work. Pathologists learn how these systems fail through natural causes, such as disease or accidental trauma. A forensic pathologist learns how the body's systems are forced to fail through unnatural means, such as gunshots and stabbings. Despite their apparently limited scope of education, forensic pathologists need to know a good bit about all the forensic sciences, as well as the natural and medical sciences. It can take 10 years of so to become a forensic pathologist. Although they are paid well by other forensic professionals' standards, they are typically paid far less than other medical doctors. The length of schooling, the nature of the work, and the relatively low pay mean that only truly dedicated can enter and excel in this demanding profession [4]. The task is to function as a medical expert for justice, not primarily to support one of the parties in the trial. Hence, the role of the forensic pathologist in the relation to the examined person is obviously completely different from the role of the clinical doctor in his/her relation to the patient, where the physician often becomes an advocate for the patient. The main role of the forensic pathologist is to practice and to mediate a scientific approach to the medical issues raised in a legal context involving death. It is inherent in its very nature that the forensic pathologist, irrespective of principle, strives to assist with impartial assessments, based on "science and tried and tested experience." [2].

3. Importance of death scene investigation before post-mortem examination

Medical expertise begins by examining the body and gathering evidence at the scene. The next step is history, physical examination, laboratory tests, and diagnosis. Providing objective evidence for the justice system and determining the timing, cause, and manner of death are the main objectives [5]. Cooperation between law and medicine was determined in 3000 B.C. in Egyptian culture. British coroner system was established at the end of the twelfth century [6]. It is very important for the forensic medicine specialist to participate in the examination of the place of death. The forensic medicine specialist can inform the investigating authority about the nature of the death, whether the circumstances are consistent with a natural death, or interpreting the amount of blood loss from a deceased person as being due to natural disease rather than injury. Not participating in death scene investigation is considered to be one of the most important mistakes in forensic medicine. The pathologists performing autopsies in the hospital who do not have time to attend death scenes or are not trained in attending death scenes should be informed about where, when, by whom, and under what circumstances the body is found. In some deaths, such as metastatic breast carcinoma, environmental factors do not contribute to death. The environment plays a role although it does not cause death in other cases: for example, a person who has significant coronary atherosclerosis dies because of dysrhythmia while shoveling snow. The findings at death scene and the photographs of the scene are critical for positional asphyxia as very few findings may be determined at the autopsy. It is very hard to determine the manner and cause of death in a 30-year-old man with a negative history and toxicology and autopsy findings of visceral congestion. But the cause and manner of death may be determined if a screwdriver is next to an electrical outlet at the decedent's house, which is in the renewal phase [7]. The investigation of the death place and then collecting the evidence material need special talent, knowledge, and ability. The manner in which a murder investigation is performed can be an important factor to determine the success of an investigation. A comprehensive examination of the site of death requires a disciplined and systematic approach to gathering observations and evidences. This should be combined with the analysis of the various observations and the relationship of the potential evidences [8]. The scene of the death should be visited in homicide, suspected homicide, and other suspicious or obscure cases, before the body is removed. Any doctor who claims to be a forensic medicine expert should accompany the police at the place of death. This duty is often formalized for forensic medicine experts who are either full-time or substantially involved in assisting the police [9]. In some cases, the scene investigation may become more important than the autopsy. A comprehensive on-scene review helps identify the cause and manner of death in a correct way [10, 11].

4. Post-mortem examination and autopsy

The key role of forensic pathologist is the examination of a corpse. "Autopsy" word is derived from the words *auto* meaning "self" and *opsy* meaning "to look at." It means "to look at one's self" or sometimes "seeing with one's own eyes." "Post mortem examination" is another alternative term for a dead body examination [4]. The earliest known forensic dissection was in Italy, at the University of Bologna in the middle of the thirteenth century. One was recorded by William of Saliceto (1210–1277) [12]. The purpose of a medicolegal autopsy is to determine the cause of death, to identify the identity of the deceased person, to estimate the post-mortem interval, and to collect evidence around the death. A medicolegal autopsy answers basic questions about "who," "what," "when," and "why" of suspicious, sudden and unnatural deaths. The identity of the deceased is usually determined by deceased's relatives. Examination of any accidental or congenital abnormality may help identify the deceased person. In situations where visual identification is difficult in mutilated or charred cases, DNA profiling and dental examination are often used to confirm the identity of the unknown person. There are some additional analyses such as post-mortem toxicology, histology, post-mortem biochemistry, immunohistochemistry, and methods of imaging (X-rays, computed tomography, magnetic resonance imaging) in modern autopsy work [4]. Though legal systems and medical conventions vary considerably from country to country, there are generally two types of autopsy: The *academic autopsy* or *clinical* is one in which the medical attendants seek to learn the extent of the disease, with the consent of relatives. The *forensic* or *medicolegal autopsy* is performed according to the instructions of the legal authority responsible for the investigation of criminal, litigious, unnatural, suspicious, or sudden deaths. The system varies from country to country, but the legal authority may be a judge, a procurator fiscal, a medical examiner, a coroner, a magistrate, or the police [9]. The formal organization of forensic medicine and the experts in forensic medicine are somewhat different in different countries. In central Europe, e.g., the medicolegal experts are recruited from a university since this has been believed to guarantee a scientific basis, independence, and impartiality. In Sweden and Finland, a national governmental authority is responsible for the administration of services in forensic medicine, whereas in the US, Canada, and several other Anglo-Saxon countries, a variety of systems are applied under the umbrella terms "coroner system" and "medical examiner system," systems that are not always easy to differentiate [2].

Author details

Kamil Hakan Dogan[1]* and Serafettin Demirci[2]

*Address all correspondence to: drhakan2000@gmail.com

1 Selcuk University, Turkey

2 Necmettin Erbakan University, Turkey

References

[1] Saukko P, Pollak S. Autopsy, procedures and standards. In: Jason P-J, editor. Encyclopedia of Forensic and Legal Medicine. Oxford: Elsevier; 2005. pp. 166-171

[2] Eriksson A. Forensic pathology. In: Freeman M, Zeegers M, editors. Forensic Epidemiology—Principles and Practice. San Diego: Academic Press; 2016. pp. 151-179

[3] Wagner SA. Death Scene Investigation—A Field Guide. Boca Raton, FL: CRC Press; 2009

[4] Houck MM. Forensic Pathology. San Diego: Academic Press; 2017

[5] Committee for the Workshop on the Medicolegal Death Investigation System. Medicolegal Death Investigation System Workshop Summary. Washington, DC: The National Academy Press; 2003

[6] Spitz WU. Medicolegal Investigation of Death: Guidelines for the Application of Pathology to Crime Investigation. 4th ed. Springfield, IL: Charles C. Thomas; 2006

[7] Lew E, Matshes E. Death scene investigation. In: Dolinak D, Matshes E, Lew E, editors. Forensic Pathology: Principles and Practice. San Diego, CA: Elsevier; 2005

[8] Horswell J. Major incident scene management. In: Payne-James J, Byard R, Corey T, Henderson C, editors. Encyclopedia of Forensic and Legal Medicine. London: Academic Press; 2005

[9] Saukko P, Knight B. The forensic autopsy. In: Saukko P, Knight B, editors. Knight's Forensic Pathology. Boca Raton: CRC Press; 2016. pp. 1-55

[10] Avis SP. An unusual suicide. The importance of the scene investigation. The American Journal of Forensic Medicine and Pathology. 1993;**142**:148-150

[11] Dix J, Ernst MF. Handbook for Death Scene Investigators. Boca Raton, FL: CRC Press; 1999

[12] Cunha F. William of Saliceto—The School of Bologna. American Journal of Surgery. 1941;**52**(1):144-149

Chapter 2

The Advancement of Postmortem Investigations in Sudden Cardiac Death

Kawthar Braysh, Raymond Zerbe,
Rosalyn Jurjus Zein, Doureid Oueidat, Jihad Hawi,
Luk Oke and Abdo Jurjus

Additional information is available at the end of the chapter

http://dx.doi.org/10.5772/intechopen.71555

Abstract

Sudden cardiac death (SCD) is a major public health issue accounting for 15–20% of all-cause deaths. Several pathologies have been associated with sudden cardiac arrest. Clinical autopsies have always contributed to invention of novel strategies for SCD prevention. One of the serious challenges that pathologists are facing is the significant decline of the overall autopsy rate. Many reasons have been associated with this change, most importantly, the evolution process in the postmortem investigation tools. However, cardiologists seem unsatisfied with the new non-invasive imaging techniques and still believe in the traditional autopsy as a gold standard in diagnosis of cardiovascular diseases. In this chapter, we focused on the importance of autopsy in the prevention of SCD by shedding a light on guidelines of minimum requirement for routine autopsy investigation of SCD (including macroscopic, histological, toxicological and molecular examination). We also gave insight into the new radiological techniques, their advantages and related diagnostic pitfalls as compared to that of conventional autopsy. Thus, providing a comprehensive understanding on the advancement of postmortem examination will help improve the minimum standards of routine autopsy practice, develop new guidelines for radiological examination and prevent the growing heterogeneity of the pathologies underlying SCD.

Keywords: autopsy practice, postmortem investigations, sudden cardiac death, coronary heart diseases, channelopathies, cardiomyopathies, non-invasive imaging techniques, toxicology

1. Introduction

Sudden cardiac death (SCD) is a term used to describe an unpredicted death of a person as a consequence of a cardiovascular event, with or without an existence of an underlying cardiac pathology [1]. It is considered as a major health problem worldwide accounting for 15–20% of all deaths [2]. This incident is associated with the development of a ventricular tachycardia (VT) which then progresses into a ventricular fibrillation (VF) and eventually asystole is followed [1]. This arrhythmic disturbance explains the rapidity of the death. SCD is generally observed in older people; nevertheless, a considerable rate has been seen in young people who are harboring an inherited cardiac lesion [2]. Identifying patients at risk of SCD is the most challenging task clinicians often face, because the great majority of SCD victims who suffer from cardiac diseases are only discovered through postmortem microscopic and macroscopic examinations when the incident of sudden death has already occurred without the presence of any previous clinical manifestations [3]. The underlying cardiac causes of SCD include coronary artery diseases (CAD), valvular heart diseases, cardiomyopathy syndromes, infiltrative diseases of the myocardium, myocarditis, infective endocarditis, inherited ion channels defects and congenital heart diseases [4, 5]. Epidemiologically, CAD is responsible for 80% of the cases of SCD, cardiomyopathies account for 10–15% of the cases, while 5–10% of SCD are caused by inherited cardiac disorders, such as coronary artery anomalies or cardiac channelopathies [6]. Coronary atherosclerosis is the most common cause of SCD in individuals aged 35 years and above, with men having a higher risk of SCD than women [4], while cardiomyopathies, especially hypertrophic cardiomyopathy (HCM), ion channels defects and coronary artery anomalies are the leading causes of SCD in adults younger than 35 years old [7]. However, in children, myocarditis and congenital heart diseases are the chief causes of SCD [4]. Besides, other non-cardiac pathologies can sometimes trigger SCD. It has been noted that patients with chronic kidney disease, obstructive sleep apnea and seizure disorders had a higher risk of developing SCD [2]. The use of medications that can have cardiac effects have been linked to many cases of SCD, such as the antipsychotic medications, some antihistamine drugs, macrolides antibiotics [8], and drugs of abuse; therefore, toxicological substances should always be considered by forensic doctors and screening tests should always be done [9]. The prevention of SCD is a field that is continuously studied [10]; however, its rate remains high despite the various preventive measures. Commonly used approaches include the use of pharmacological interventions and implantable cardioverter-defibrillator (ICD) [10]. An important measure for prevention is to identify those at risk of a SCD, Framingham risk score is a commonly used method, it is recommended as a routine screening method in males in their 40s and in postmenopausal women. It calculates an individual risk of CAD substrate based on multiple variables like age, sex, smoking, blood pressure, LDL levels, body mass index (BMI) and diabetes; consequently, labeling people who might require preventive interventions. The role of ECG in identifying future victims is still uncertain; however, its role in prediction of SCD in those with identified genetic arrhythmic disease is clear, mostly in Long QT Syndrome. Actually the degree of QT interval prolongation positively correlates with the risk [11]. Additionally, screening young athletes for a hidden cardiac pathology has become increasingly demanded before starting physical activity, as SCD can be precipitated during sport, and ECG is one of the most commonly first-line screening tool along with physical examination that are encouraged to be practiced methods in young individuals before engaging in sport activities.

Positive results are followed by non-invasive imaging techniques like echo, CT, MRI among others or invasive ones like angiography and electrophysiological studies [12].

2. Management of a SCD from the forensic angle

The practice in postmortem examination involves a detailed patient and family history, questioning regarding the patient's condition before death, as well as, macroscopic and histological studies of the heart with investigations of other organs to exclude non-cardiac causes of death, followed by a genetic testing of a blood sample. Then a complete clinical and genetic testing is done on family members who are at risk [13]. Generally, the autopsy protocols of SCD start with a macroscopic study of the heart, if the cause is identified no further testing is required. However, a negative macroscopic testing is followed by either a histological or a genetic testing depending on the victim's age. Histological testing is the next step in victims more than 30 years old with a negative macroscopic study, a positive test requires no further steps, while a negative one is followed by a genetic study. On the other hand, genetic testing is done as the next step on victims less than 30 years old with a negative macroscopic study [14]. When dealing with a heart autopsy, several steps are required; the pericardium should be checked for abnormalities, the pulmonary arteries should be examined for the presence of an embolus, and the patterns of origins of coronary arteries and their distributions are thoroughly investigated to determine a possible luminal obstruction. In addition, the ventricles are studied to determine chamber size, the valve, wall thickness, and the presence of zones of new or old infracts [15] and to assess for the intactness of the papillary muscles and the chordae tendineae [9]. The left and right atria should be opened and their respective cavities should be thoroughly investigated and the assessment of the patency of the foramen ovale is followed [9]. Once the heart is evacuated from blood, multiple measurements are taken including the heart weight, its wall thickness and its dimensions [9]. Histological investigations are carried by examining the obtained tissues after staining with hematoxylin and eosin and Masson trichrome stain [16]. A negative autopsy is defined as the absence of any identifiable structural heart defect, with a negative histological and toxicological testing. The presence of a negative autopsy is a strong indicator of the presence of an inherited cardiac arrhythmic disease, this usually require a genetic testing on the victim, a process commonly termed as the molecular autopsy [13]. While the routine postmortem examination still possesses an essential role in the investigation of SCD, nowadays, the use of non-invasive imaging techniques such as multi-detector computed tomography (MDCT), CT angiography, and cardiac magnetic resonance imaging (MRI) [17] has shown its significance in diagnosing structural causes of cardiac death. It has also overcome some families' religious objections [13].

3. Autopsy examination for SCD

3.1. Macroscopic studies

Macroscopic examination of the heart helps in the identification of structural causes of SCD. Autopsy findings in SCD due to CAD include an alteration in the plaque structure such as thrombus formation or plaque disruption such as fissuring or hemorrhage. Plaque rupture is the primary event that initiates the process of thrombus formation leading to acute coronary syndrome and SCD [18, 19]. Stenosis of more than 75% of the arterial lumen has been noted in a great proportion of individuals who have survived from a sudden cardiac arrest [18]. The development of collateral circulation in chronic ischemic heart disease patients has a protective role as it provides blood to areas distal to a stenotic region [18]. Hypertrophic cardiomyopathy (HCM), an autosomal dominant disease which occurs due to mutations in genes coding for sarcomere proteins, can be present in SCD of young individuals. Moreover, mutations in a-tropomyosin and beta myosin heavy gene have the greatest risk of causing SCD [18]. Morphologically, it is characterized by left ventricular (LV) wall thickness, asymmetrical septal hypertrophy and mid-ventricular obstruction. On the other hand, dilated cardiomyopathy, which has both a genetic and non-genetic components, is associated with dilation of the left and right ventricles, thrombi may be observed in the cardiac chambers, and wall thickness may be increased or decreased [20]. Arrhythmogenic right ventricular dysplasia is another type of cardiomyopathy that can be associated with SCD; it is heritable disease with an autosomal dominant pattern whose genetic mutation has been localized on chromosome 1. Exercise is a common trigger of arrhythmia in these patients. Cardiac atrophy is seen in autopsy as a result of myocyte apoptosis [18]. Myocarditis, an inflammatory process in the myocardium, is a common cause of SCD; autopsy can show ventricular dilation with a mottled appearance along with scaring, fibrosis and minor coronary occlusion [21]. Infective endocarditis is another infectious cardiac disease which can induce SCD due to many causes. On gross examination of the heart, one can detect the presence of a vegetation on the infected valve, erosion of the underlying tissue, the chordae tendineae may be disrupted resulting in their rupture [5]. Congenital heart diseases occupy a high rank in the causes of SCD in children, with coarctation of the aorta (CoA) and transposition of the great vessels in the forefront [22]. In coarctation of the aorta, stenosis is observed proximal to the ductus arteriosus and distal to the left subclavian artery, this impedes the normal flow of blood through the aorta. Simultaneous cardiac anomalies can also accompany CoA, bicuspid aortic valve is being the most common, therefore, a close examination of the heart is required [23, 24]. In transposition of the great arteries an atypical origin of the arteries is seen at the base of the heart [23].

3.2. Microscopic investigations

In cases related to myocardial infarction in SCD, it is important to highlight the fact that histological defects differ based on the date of infarction [25]. Routine Hematoxylin and Eosin (H&E) stain will detect signs of cellular death and necrosis after 6 to 8 hours of ischemia. These signs include myofiber eosinophilia, elongation of sarcomeres and nuclei, wavy fibers, interstitial edema and contraction band. Therefore, if SCD occurs in early ischemia before this time frame, these changes will not be detected neither histologically nor macroscopically. From this perspective, many studies have suggested the role of histochemical and immunohistochemical staining in the detection of early ischemia. C5b-C9 complex, which is the last creation of the activated complement cascade that forms the membrane attack complex (MAC), is a specific marker for early necrosis. Other markers being tested include complement proteins like C1, C3, C8, C9 and inflammatory mediators such as CD15, IL-1, IL-6, TNF-, IL-15, IL-8, MCP-1,

CD18 as well as tryptase which have shown positive results in early hours of ischemia. It has been documented by several studies on human as well on animal models that myoglobin and troponins especially troponin T are lost during the early stages of myocardial ischemia and observing their absence using immunohistochemical staining is a useful test in detecting early infarction [26]. Moreover, Microscopic findings in HCM include myocardial fiber disarray and myocytes hypertrophy which is associated with 4 fold increase in cell and nuclear size. An abnormal thickening of the coronary arterioles can also be noted [27, 28]. Identifying myocarditis as a cause in SCD is often a difficult process as the microscopic findings are not always accurate. Based on the principal type of infiltrating inflammatory cells, it can be classified into lymphocytic, neutrophilic, eosinophilic and giant cell types. Diffuse inflammation with myocytes necrosis and conduction system damage is the microscopic findings that have the highest probability of diagnosing myocarditis as a cause of death [21]. Histologically, the classic findings of vegetation in infective endocarditis are tissue infiltration of neutrophils and fibrin deposition along with the implicated bacteria can be identified using gram stain. In rare cases, a vegetative embolus may lodge in a coronary artery which can be the cause of SCD, in these circumstances the embolus has the same characteristic microscopic picture of the original vegetation [5]. The hearts of patients who suffered from arrhythmogenic right ventricular dysplasia exhibit microscopic features of fat infiltrating the myocardium, fibrofatty replacement along with patchy areas of myocarditis [18]. In cases of rare cardiomyopathies such as those associated with mitochondrial and storage diseases, an electron microscopy is usually required [9].

3.3. Toxicological studies in SCD

Toxicological examination is also mandatory and scientifically a useful tool to determine the causes of SCD. Toxicological analysis can identify if sudden death is triggered by administration of toxic substances. This latter could be prescribed and non-prescribed medications, illicit or recreational drugs that are widely abused by athletes or young individuals [29]. The rising use of recreational drugs among adolescents and young adults is a common phenomenon seen worldwide. Cocaine is a well-known stimulant drug of abuse that is linked to cardiac death, along with amphetamines. Their respective mechanisms of action are similar as they both cause the release of catecholamines such as norepinephrine, dopamine and serotonin leading to coronary vasospasm and thrombus formation. This combination of adverse effects can lead to myocardial ischemia and infarction in the absence of atherosclerosis [30]. Cannabis is another commonly abused drug that it is becoming more legalized in many countries. Although its associated side effects are typically low, it causes cardiovascular side effects. Cannabis raises the blood pressure and heart rate and can induce arrhythmia and myocardial ischemia [31]. In rare instances, the occurrence of SCD in acute cannabis intoxication has been described. It has been also demonstrated that some drugs have been strongly associated with SCD including the antipsychotic medications. Their proposed mechanism of action is associated with the development of myocarditis and the ability to cause a prolongation in QT interval which then progresses into a life-threatening arrhythmia [32]. Referring to the guidelines adapted by the Society of Forensic Toxicologists and the American Academy of Forensic Sciences [33], multiple samples should be studied including heart blood, peripheral blood collected from the femoral vein, urine or bile. Hair from the back of the scalp or pubic hair should also be used for doing toxicological analysis [9]. Therefore, toxicological analysis is to be considered as a cornerstone in postmortem studies, in order to screen for potential ingestion of medications that are linked to cardiac side effects and to look for possible intoxication of drug of abuse.

3.4. Molecular studies of cardiac autopsy

The causes of SCD, which remain unidentified after complete autopsy procedures including the macroscopic, microscopic and toxicological examinations, are classified as sudden arrhythmic death syndromes. At this point, molecular testing plays a critical role in identifying the SCD in victims of structurally normal heart. Sudden arrhythmic death syndromes (SAD) are defined as genetic heart diseases that cause sudden death in young people that apparently look healthy. They are classified into two subcategories: (1) cardiac channelopathies that are caused by mutations affecting different cardiac membrane channels such as Long QT syndrome (LQTS), Short QT syndrome (SQTS), and Brugada syndrome (BrS) or cellular structure resulting in dysregulated Ca2+ release including catecholaminergic polymorphic ventricular tachycardia (CPVT) [34, 35], and (2) cardiomyopathies such as hypertrophic cardiomyopathy (HCM), dilated cardiomyopathy (DCM), arrhythmogenic cardiomyopathy (AC) and others. At least 64 genes have been identified to cause cardiomyopathies syndromes [36]. Although cardiomyopathies usually depict distinct structural alterations on autopsy, some cases, especially in children may present a structurally normal heart [14]. This is in contrast with inherited diseases of conduction (LQTS, BrS) that do not show any structural abnormalities on autopsy, making it a challenging task to the pathologist to detect the causes of SCD [13]. LQTS are characterized by QT interval on ECG that leads to the development of syncope and arrhythmic disturbances which are directly linked to SCD such as torsade de pointes. The majority of LQTS is autosomal dominant. There are 14 types of LQTS that have been identified based on the gene involved and location of mutation. For instance, KCNQ1 mutation is associated with the development of LQTS1, KCNH2 with LQTS2 and SCN5A with LQTS3. It has been indicated that LQTS1 is triggered by exercising such as swimming, LQRTS2 by sudden loud noises such alarms, while LQTS3 occurs during sleep or at rest [34, 35]. SQTS is considered as the severest condition of cardiac channelopathies. It is characterized by K+ channel gain-of-function mutations. Additionally, BrS also can cause SCD in 4–12% of the cases. It is characterized by genetic mutation targeting Na+ channels [34, 35]. Its ECG pattern is associated with an elevated ST segment that develops either unexpectedly or as a result of the administration of sodium channel blockers [37]. BrS is associated with monomorphic ventricular tachycardia that usually occurs during sleep, at rest or in case of severe fever. Unlike LQTS, data available on gene specific prognostication and risk stratification are very limited in the case of SQTS and BrS [34, 35]. On the other side, CPVT is a significant cause of sudden unexplained death. It is most common among young males. Individuals with CPVT show normal resting ECG with functionally and structurally normal heart. They can develop syncope as a result of physical activity, a strong emotional stimulus or SD secondary to Catecholaminergic Polymorphic Ventricular Tachycardia (CPVT). The current genetic techniques allow us to unmask the etiology behind SCD. The detection of an underlying genetic mutation facilitates the process of detecting people at risk in order to take preventive measures [14]. Polymerase chain reaction (PCR) is one example of the postmortem molecular investigation techniques. It involves the amplification of a specific DNA sequence by an enzymatic reaction. It consists of multiple rounds of heat denaturation, annealing of primers and a DNA polymerase dependent chain elongation [3] of a blood sample collected in postmortem exam for genetic testing or from a fixed tissue sample [38]. This molecular technique, could detect mutations in the genes coding for potassium channels (KCNQ1, KCNH2), sodium channels (SCN5A), and the RYR2 gene which causes tachycardia (CPVT) [39, 40]. The provided table (**Table 1**) shows the 90 implicated genes for the most common inherited

---

A. Cardiomyopathies

a. Dilated cardiomyopathy

- ATP- binding cassette, subfamily C (CFTR/MRP), member 9 [ABCC9]
- Bcl2-associated athanogene 3 [BAG3]
- Desmin [DES]
- Dystrophin muscular dystrophy [DMD]
- Emerin (Emery-Dreifuss muscular dystrophy) [EMD]
- Eyes absent homolog 4 (Drosophila) [EYA4]
- Fukuyama-type congenital muscular dystrophy (fukutin)1 [FCMD]
- Integrin-linked kinase ILK
- Lamin A/C [LMNA]
- Myopalladin [MYPN]
- Presenilin 1 [PSEN1]
- Presenilin 2 [PSEN2]
- RNA-binding motif protein 20 [RBM20]
- Sarcoglycan, d (dystrophin-associated glycoprotein) [SGCD]
- Tafazzin [TAZ]

b. Hypertrophic cardiomyopathy

- Calreticulin 3 [CALR3]
- Frataxin [FXN]
- GATA-binding protein 4 GLA galactosidase, a [GATA4]
- Jagged 1 [JAG1]
- Junctophilin 2 [JPH2]
- Myosin, light chain 2, regulatory, cardiac, slow [MYL2]
- Myosin, light chain 3, alkali; ventricular, skeletal, slow [MYL3]
- Myomesin 1, 185 kDa [MYOM1]
- Myozenin 2 [MYOZ2]
- Protein kinase, AMP-activated, 2 noncatalytic subunit [PRKAG2]
- Protein tyrosine phosphatase, nonreceptor type 11 [PTPN11]
- V-raf-1 murine leukemia viral oncogene homolog 1 [RAF1]

c. Arrhythmogenic cardiomyopathy

- Desmocollin 2 [DSC2]

- Desmoglein 2 [DSG2]
- Desmoplakin [DSP]
- Junction plakoglobin [JUP]
- Phospholamban [PLN]
- Transforming growth factor, [b3 TGFB3]
- Transmembrane protein 43 [TMEM43]

B. Channelopathies

a. Long QT syndrome (LQTS)

- A kinase (PRKA) anchor protein (yotiao) 9 [AKAP9]
- Ankyrin 2 [ANK2]
- Calmodulin 2 [CALM2]
- Caveolin 3 [CAV3]
- Potassium voltage-gated channel, Isk-related family, member 1 [KCNE1]
- Potassium voltage-gated channel, Isk-related family, member 2 [KCNE2]
- Potassium voltage-gated channel, subfamily H (eag-related), member 2 [KCNH2]
- Potassium inwardly rectifying channel, subfamily J, member 2 [KCNJ2]
- Potassium inwardly rectifying channel, subfamily J, member 5 [KCNJ5]
- Potassium voltage-gated channel, KQT-like subfamily, member 1 [KCNQ1]
- Sodium channel, voltage-gated, type IV, b [SCN4B]
- Syntrophin, a 1 [SNTA1]

b. Brugada syndrome (BrS)

- Calcium channel, voltage-dependent, a 2/d subunit 1 [CACNA2D1]
- Calcium channel, voltage-dependent, b 2 subunit [CACNB2]
- Glycerol-3-phosphate dehydrogenase 1–like [GPD1L]
- Calcium channel, voltage-dependent, b 2 subunit [CACNB2]
- Hyperpolarization-activated cyclic nucleotide–gated potassium channel 4 [HCN4]
- Potassium voltage-gated channel, Shal-related family, member 3 [KCND3]
- Potassium voltage-gated channel, Isk-related family, member 3 [KCNE3]
- Potassium inwardly rectifying channel, subfamily J, member 8 [KCNJ8]
- RAN guanine nucleotide release factor [RANGRF]
- Sodium channel, voltage-gated, type I, b [SCN1B]
- Sodium channel, voltage-gated, type III, b [SCN3B]

c. Catecholaminergic polymorphic ventricular tachycardia (CPVT)

- Triadin [TRDN]
- Ryanodine receptor 2 (cardiac) [RYR2]
- Calmodulin 1 [CALM1]

Table 1. Common genetic mutations associated with inherited cardiac diseases.

channelopathies and cardiomyopathies. On the other hand, next whole-exome sequencing (WES) is a new available genetic testing technique that may become an important part in post mortem studies in the future [41]. This technique allows us to study the whole genetic library of an individual DNA sample, which is more effective and better than studying a specific gene. To ensure that an adequate WES testing is being performed, it is recommended to use about 5 to 10 ml of blood collected for DNA testing or 5 g of tissue extracted from the heart or spleen [36]. Next Generation Sequencing (NGS) is also new available genetic sequencing technique for detecting channelopathies associated-mutations, which has a sensitivity of 72% for LQTS cases [42]. Thus, molecular autopsy has taken a major part in revealing the gene mutations associated with cardiac channelopathies and other inherited heart diseases and provided evidence for the importance of cardiological assessment for first-degree family members after SCD in order to prevent future tragedies [43].

4. Non-invasive imaging techniques in SCD

Minimally invasive or non-invasive autopsy methods have been recently developed and implemented to substitute clinically invasive autopsy. Computed tomography (CT) and Magnetic resonance imaging (MRI) are two imaging modalities that are increasingly used in post-mortem investigation of SCD [17]. Cardiac MRI is considered as reference for ventricular function assessment and risk stratification measurement [44]. The introduction of post mortem computed tomography coronory angiography (PMCTA) has also been shown to be a very powerful tool in demonstrating the patency of the coronaries, identifying stenotic defects in the coronaries and guiding sampling for histology. It enables the detection and documentation of coronary artery calcification. On the other hand, post mortem magnetic resonance (PMMR) has shown its significant diagnostic ability in postmortem autopsy, mainly in assessing the heart valves, myocardial wall thickness, and ischemic changes [45]. Despite the great advantages of these techniques, one adverse event is thrombi dislodgement and the inability to differentiate between pre and post mortem thrombi. Moreover, their high cost and the need of well-trained physicians in this radiological field is also another pitfall [17]. Recent studies have been conducted by Ampazoni et al. on the PMMR to assess its importance as an alternative or an adjuvant to traditional autopsy. Results show that cardiac parameters measured by PMMR may differ from the measures obtained by autopsy and forensic pathologists should be aware of these differences. Additionally, there is no conventional value for wall thickness and valves circumferences when measured by PMMR, thus further research is required to get cutoff values [45].

5. Conventional autopsy vs. non-invasive imaging examination

Several studies have reinforced the importance of autopsy in investigating the cause behind sudden unexplained death, the nature of cardiac disease in case of SCD, the underlying mechanism, whether it is arrhythmic or mechanical or it originates from genetic mutations, and the possibility of illicit drug abuse [9]. Autopsy is also of vital importance in providing accurate epidemiological data and data for evaluating of the quality of care, identifying and elucidating new pathological findings, evaluating new medical interventions, improving post-marketing surveillance for adverse effects of drugs, devices, and procedures, improving cardiovascular diseases research and offering powerful tools for education [46, 47]. However, many pitfalls and limitations are encountered with the use of non- forensic autopsies in modern medicine. One of these major challenges is the significant decline of autopsy rate, wherein autopsies are performed after less than 10% of all U.S death. In fact, studies have shown that clinicians and pathologists have no more incentives to perform the autopsy and they are focusing on the new imaging approaches [48]. The most significant consequence of this shift is the increased frequency of clinical diagnostic discrepancies of class I and class II. These errors include the misdiagnosed or undiagnosed conditions that likely lead to patients death (class I) or do not affect the survival (class II), excluding the over or delayed diagnosis [49]. The autopsy rate has declined over the last decades for a number of reasons. The lack of the financial support and direct reimbursement of the pathologists on their services is the major driving force to this decline. The change in economic landscape has led both the public and the private healthcare sectors to increase focus on cost control [48]. For instance, the lack of funding from insurance companies and other payers for advocating postmortem genetic testing made the molecular autopsy less frequent or less practiced by forensic pathologists [47]. More importantly and in the line of autopsy practice, pathologists are facing difficulties in the lack of standardizations of sudden death coding and the variation of SD definition among different regions and countries that hinder their task in determining the precise cause of sudden death. Additionally, the inconsistency in the routine autopsy practice among hospitals, university medical centers and forensic medicine institutes has also been a central issue. This is strongly associated with the inaccurate autopsy reports that are difficult to interpret and do not precisely resolve the diagnostic questions. It has been demonstrated that the quality of the autopsy report was judged to be satisfactory in 52%, good or excellent in a further 23%; but was poor or unacceptable in 26% [50], suggesting that only half of the autopsies are satisfactory and have answered the basic clinical question over the cause of death. But the much more important observed phenomenon is the criteria variation of report formulation. As mentioned, part of the autopsy reports are categorized as good which means that the autopsy report fulfills its main purpose of documenting the cause of death but without much elaboration or details, while unacceptable reports are those that appear to be evidently wrong [50]. For this purpose, the Association for European Cardiovascular Pathology has developed guidelines for autopsy investigation for SCD cases. Basso C et al., have described in details autopsy procedures that should be followed in order to represent the minimum standard that is required in the routine autopsy practice for the adequate assessment of SCD including standard gross examination of the heart, histological sampling, toxicology and molecular examination [9]. Similarly for the case of autopsy reports, there should be nationally uniform criteria and standards for reporting autopsy findings. This includes the diagnostic level of autopsy investigation and the definition of what a postmortem examination comprises. They should also be standardized in topics according to a diagnostic hierarchy that takes into consideration both the logical sequence of events that led to death and the organs involved [50]. On the other side, the introduction of the alternative postmortem imaging techniques has recently replaced to a great extent the use of clinical autopsy. These radiological examination tools have become more feasible for the physicians so that they are no more obliged to ask for consent from victim's next of kin which is often refused

http://dx.doi.org/10.5772/intechopen.71555

by bereaved families due to cultural and religious objections. Forensic specialists have proved the high diagnostic performance of these postmortem imaging tools in forensic studies. Nevertheless, cardiologists seem unsatisfied with the diagnosis reports of these techniques and they find it hard to replace the conventional autopsy. They consider that the diagnostic accuracy of the imaging tools alone is insufficient for detecting the exact cause of SCD and still believe in autopsy as the gold standard. Misinterpretation is one of the major pitfalls of radiological examination. Radiological findings cannot sometimes distinguish the presence of possible artifacts. These artifacts could be incidental and unrelated to the cause of death [51]. Sometimes postmortem changes can also limit specific imaging diagnosis and interfere with the radiological results such as in thrombosis [52]. Additionally, there are still no gold standards that currently exist for postmortem radiological examination of cardiovascular pathologies.

6. Conclusion

Postmortem radiology is a promising approach but currently cannot replace conventional autopsy. In brief, we can conclude that advances in diagnostic technology have not reduced the value of the autopsy and the goal-directed autopsy remains a vital component in the assurance of good medical care [53]. More studies and research are still warranted to establish the validity and limitations of postmortem radiology in the identification of SCD. In the meantime, the use of non-invasive imaging approach should accompany and complement conventional autopsy procedures in order to enhance a significant advancement in the postmortem investigation of SCD (**Figure 1**).

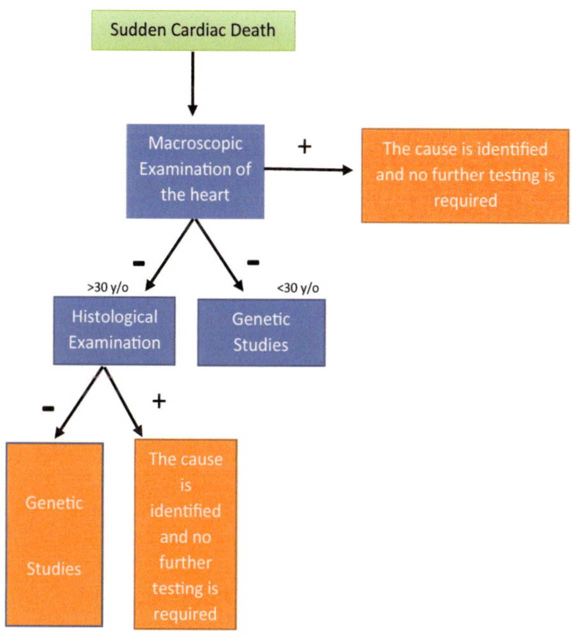

Figure 1. The appropriate steps when dealing with sudden cardiac Death.

Author details

Kawthar Braysh[1], Raymond Zerbe[1], Rosalyn Jurjus Zein[2], Doureid Oueidat[1], Jihad Hawi[3], Luk Oke[4] and Abdo Jurjus[1]*

*Address all correspondence to: aj00@aub.edu.lb

1 Department of Anatomy, Cell Biology and Physiological Sciences, American University of Beirut, Beirut, Lebanon

2 Department of Anatomy and Regenerative Biology, School of Medicine and Health Sciences, George Washington University, Washington DC, USA

3 Department of Biomedical Sciences, Faculty of Medicine and Medical Sciences, Balamand University, Lebanon

4 American Center for Investigative Cardiology Silver Spring, Maryland, USA

References

[1] Lopshire JC, Zipes DP. Sudden cardiac death: Better understanding of risks, mechanisms, and treatment. Circulation. 2006;**114**(11):1134-1136. DOI: 10.1161/CIRCULATIONAHA.106.647933

[2] Hayashi M, Shimizu W, Albert CM. The spectrum of epidemiology underlying sudden cardiac death. Circulation Research. 2015;**116**(12):1887-1906. DOI: 10.1161/CIRCRESAHA.116.304521

[3] Basso C, Calabrese F, Corrado D, Thiene G. Postmortem diagnosis in sudden cardiac death victims: Macroscopic, microscopic and molecular findings. Cardiovascular Research. 2001;**50**(2):290-300

[4] Virmani R, Burke AP, Farb A. Sudden cardiac death. Cardiovascular Pathology. 2001;**10**(5):211-218

[5] Castelli JB, Almeida G, Siciliano RF. Sudden death in infective endocarditis. The Journal Autopsy and Case Reports. 2016;**6**(3):17-22

[6] Wilhelm M, Bolliger SA, Bartsch C, Fokstuen S, et al. Sudden cardiac death in forensic medicine – Swiss recommendations for a multidisciplinary approach. Swiss Medical Weekly. 2015;**w14129**:145. DOI: 10.4414/smw.2015.14129

[7] Finocchiaro G, Papadakis M, Sharma S, Sheppard M. Sudden cardiac death. European Heart Journal. 2017;**38**(17):1280-1282. DOI: 10.1093/eurheartj/ehx194

[8] Glassman AH, Bigger JT Jr. Antipsychotic drugs: Prolonged QTc interval, torsade de pointes, and sudden death. The American Journal of Psychiatry. 2001;**158**(11):1774-1782. DOI: 10.1176/appi.ajp.158.11.1774

[9] Basso C, Burke M, Fornes P, Gallagher PJ, de Gouveia RH, Sheppard M, Thiene G, van der Wal A, Association for European Cardiovascular Pathology. Guidelines for autopsy investigation of sudden cardiac death. Virchows Archiv. 2008 Jan;**452**(1):11-18. Epub 2007 Oct 20. DOI: 10.1007/s00428-007-0505-5

[10] Fishman GI, Chugh SS, Dimarco JP, Albert CM, et al. Sudden cardiac death prediction and prevention: Report from a National Heart, Lung, and Blood Institute and Heart Rhythm Society workshop. Circulation. 2010 Nov 30;**122**(22):2335-2348. DOI: 10.1161/CIRCULATIONAHA.110.976092

[11] Wellens HJ, Schwartz PJ, Lindemans FW, Buxton AE, et al. Risk stratification for sudden cardiac death: Current status and challenges for the future. European Heart Journal. 2014;**35**(25):1642-1651. DOI: 10.1093/eurheartj/ehu176

[12] Thiene G, Corrado D, Rigato I, Basso C. Why and how to support screening strategies to prevent sudden death in athletes. Cell and Tissue Research. 2012;**348**(2):315-318. DOI: 10.1007/s00441-012-1398-4

[13] Semsarian C, Ingles J, Wilde AA. Sudden cardiac death in the young: The molecular autopsy and a practical approach to surviving relatives. European Heart Journal. 2015; **36**(21):1290-1296. DOI: 10.1093/eurheartj/ehv063

[14] Goldman AM, Behr ER, Semsarian C, Bagnall RD, Sisodiya S, Cooper PN. Sudden unexpected death in epilepsy genetics: Molecular diagnostics and prevention. Epilepsia. 2016;**57**:17-25. DOI: 10.1111/epi.13232

[15] Bailey D. Guidelines on Autopsy Practice: Sudden Death with Likely Cardiac Pathology; 2015

[16] Di Gioia CR, Autore C, Romeo DM, Ciallella C, et al. Sudden cardiac death in younger adults: Autopsy diagnosis as a tool for preventive medicine. Human Pathology. 2006;**37**(7):794-801. DOI: 10.1016/j.humpath.2006.03.008

[17] Michaud K, Grabherr S, Jackowski C, Bollmann MD, Doenz F, Mangin P. Postmortem imaging of sudden cardiac death. International Journal of Legal Medicine. 2014 Jan;**128**(1):127-137. DOI: 10.1007/s00414-013-0819-6

[18] Zipes DP, Wellens HJ. Sudden cardiac death. Circulation. 1998;**98**(21):2334-2351

[19] Carrizo S, Peinado RP, Sanchez-Recalde A, Ruiz-Garcia J, et al. Clinical and angiographic characteristics of patients with acute coronary syndrome associated with sudden cardiac death. Hellenic Journal of Cardiology. 2015;**56**(2):136-141

[20] Hashimura H, Kimura F, Ishibashi-Ueda H, Morita Y, et al. Radiologic-pathologic correlation of primary and secondary cardiomyopathies: MR imaging and histopathologic findings in hearts from autopsy and transplantation. Radiographics. 2017;**37**(3):719-736. DOI: 10.1148/rg.2017160082

[21] Li L, Zhang Y, Burke A, Xue A, et al. Demographic, clinical and pathological features of sudden deaths due to myocarditis: Results from a state-wide population-based autopsy study. Forensic Science International. 2017;**272**:81-86. DOI: 10.1016/j.forsciint.2016.12.037

[22] Lynge TH, Jeppesen AG, Winkel BG, Sondergaard L, Risgaard B, Tfelt-Hansen J. Decline in incidence of sudden cardiac death caused by congenital heart disease after implementation of nationwide prenatal ultrasound screening: A nationwide study. Circulation. 2016;**134**(1). DOI: A14270

[23] Erickson KL. An approach to the examination of the fetal congenitally malformed heart at autopsy. Journal of Fetal Medicine. 2015;**2**(3):135-141

[24] Sadeghpour A, Alizadehasl A, Mahdavi M. Coarctation of the aorta. In: Sadeghpour A, Kyavar M, Alizadehasl A, editors. Comprehensive Approach to Adult Congenital Heart Disease. London: Springer; 2014, p. 289-297

[25] Takahashi Y, Sano R, Takahashi K, Kominato Y, et al. Use of postmortem coronary computed tomography angiography with water-insoluble contrast medium to detect stenosis of the left anterior descending artery in a case of sudden death. Legal Medicine (Tokyo). 2016;**19**:47-51. DOI: 10.1016/j.legalmed.2016.02.003

[26] Mondello C, Cardia L, Ventura-Spagnolo E. Immunohistochemical detection of early myocardial infarction: A systematic review. International Journal of Legal Medicine. 2017;**131**(2):411-421. DOI: 10.1007/s00414-016-1494-1

[27] Sabater-Molina M, Pérez-Sánchez I, Hernández Del Rincón JP, Gimeno JR. Genetics of hypertrophic cardiomyopathy: A review of current state. Clinical Genetics. 2017. DOI: 10.1111/cge.13027

[28] Tavora F, Cresswell N, Li L, Ripple M, Fowler D, Burke A. Morphologic features of exertional versus nonexertional sudden death in patients with hypertrophic cardiomyopathy. The American Journal of Cardiology. 2010;**105**(4):532-537. DOI: 10.1016/j.amjcard.2009.10.022

[29] Kennedy MC, Lawrence C. Anabolic steroid abuse and cardiac death. The Medical Journal of Australia. 1993;**158**(5):346-348

[30] Fischbach P. The role of illicit drug use in sudden death in the young. Cardiology in the Young. 2017;**27**(S1):S75-S79. DOI: 10.1017/S1047951116002274

[31] Hartung B, Kauferstein S, Ritz-Timme S, Daldrup T. Sudden unexpected death under acute influence of cannabis. Forensic Science International. 2014;**237**:e11-e13. DOI: 10.1016/j.forsciint.2014.02.001

[32] Straus SM, Bleumink GS, Dieleman JP, van der Lei J, et al. Antipsychotics and the risk of sudden cardiac death. Archives of Internal Medicine. 2004;**164**(12):1293-1297

[33] SOFT/AAFS Forensic Laboratory Guidelines. 2006. Available from: http://www.soft tox.org/files/Guidelines_2006_Final.pdf

[34] Behere SP, Weindling SN. Inherited arrhythmias: The cardiac channelopathies. Annals of Pediatric Cardiology. 2015;**8**(3):210-220. DOI: 10.4103/0974-2069.164695

[35] Schwartz PJ, Ackerman MJ, GeorgeJr AL, Wilde AM. Impact of genetics on the clinical management of channelopathies. Journal of the American College of Cardiology. 2013;**62**(3):169-180. DOI: doi.org/10.1016/j.jacc.2013.04.044

[36] Loporcaro CG, Tester DJ, Maleszewski JJ, Kruisselbrink T, Ackerman MJ. Confirmation of cause and manner of death via a comprehensive cardiac autopsy including whole exome next-generation sequencing. Archives of Pathology & Laboratory Medicine. 2014;**138**(8):1083-1089. DOI: 10.5858/arpa.2013-0479-SA

[37] Lahrouchi N, Behr ER, Bezzina1 CR. Next-generation sequencing in post-mortem genetic testing of young sudden cardiac death cases. Frontiers in Cardiovascular Medicine. 2016;**3**:13. DOI: 10.3389/fcvm.2016.00013

[38] Bagnall RD, Ingles J, Yeates L, Berkovic SF, Semsarian C. Exome sequencing-based molecular autopsy of formalin-fixed paraffin-embedded tissue after sudden death. Genetics in Medicine. 2017. DOI: 10.1038/gim.2017.15

[39] Semsarian C, Ingles J. Molecular autopsy in victims of inherited arrhythmias. Journal of Arrhythmia. 2016 Oct;**32**(5):359-365

[40] Bagnall RD, Semsarian C. Role of the molecular autopsy in the investigation of sudden cardiac death. Progress in Pediatric Cardiology. 2017;**45**:17-23. DOI: doi.org/10.1016/j.ppedcard.2017.02.005

[41] Sanchez O, Campuzano O, Fernández-Falgueras A, Sarquella-Brugada G, et al. Natural and undetermined sudden death: Value of post-mortem genetic investigation. PLoS One. 2016 Dec 8;**11**(12):e0167358. DOI: 10.1371/journal.pone.0167358

[42] Lieve KV, Williams L, Daly A, Richard G, Bale S, Macaya D, Chung WK. Results of genetic testing in 855 consecutive unrelated patients referred for long QT syndrome in a clinical laboratory. Genetic Testing and Molecular Biomarkers. 2013;**17**(7):553-561. DOI: 10.1089/gtmb.2012.0118

[43] Torkamani A, Muse ED, Spencer EG, Rueda M, Wagner GN, Lucas JR, Topol EJ. Molecular autopsy for sudden unexpected death. Journal of the American Medical Association. 2016;**316**(14):1492-1494. DOI: 10.1001/jama.2016.11445

[44] Sparrow PJ, Merchant N, Provost YL, Doyle DJ, Nguyen ET, Paul NS. CT and MR imaging findings in patients with acquired heart disease at risk for sudden cardiac death. Radiographics. 2009;**29**(3):805-823. DOI: 10.1148/rg.293085715

[45] Ampanozi G, Hatch GM, Flach PM, Thali MJ, Ruder TD. Postmortem magnetic resonance imaging: Reproducing typical autopsy heart measurements. Legal Medicine (Tokyo). 2015;**17**(6):493-498. DOI: 10.1016/j.legalmed.2015.10.008

[46] Saad R, Yamada AT, Pereira da Rosa FH, Gutierrez PS, Mansur AJ. Comparison between clinical and autopsy diagnoses in a cardiology hospital. Heart. 2007;**93**(11):1414-1419

[47] Shojania KG, Burton EC. The vanishing nonforensic autopsy. The New England Journal of Medicine. 2008;**358**(9):873-875. DOI: 10.1056/NEJMp0707996

[48] Nemetz PN, Tanglos E, Sands LP, Fisher WP Jr, Newman WP 3rd, Burton EC. Attitudes toward the autopsy–an 8-state survey. MedGenMed. 2006 Sep 21;**8**(3):80

[49] Graber ML. The incidence of diagnostic error in medicine. BMJ Quality and Safety. 2013 Oct;**22**(Suppl 2):ii21-ii27. DOI: 10.1136/bmjqs-2012-001615

[50] A Report of the National Confidential Enquiry into Patient Outcome and Death (2006) – The Coroner's Autopsy: Do we Deserve Better?. Available from: http://www.ncepod.org.uk/2006Report/Downloads/Coronial%20Autopsy%20Report%202006.pdf

[51] Shriki JE, Shinbane J, Lee C, Khan AR, Burns N, Hindoyan A, Wilcox A. Incidental myocardial infarct on conventional nongated CT: A review of the spectrum of findings with gated CT and cardiac MRI correlation. AJR. American Journal of Roentgenology. 2012;**198**(3):496-504. DOI: 10.2214/AJR.11.7683

[52] Roberts IS, Benamore RE, Benbow EW, Lee SH, et al. Post-mortem imaging as an alternative to autopsy in the diagnosis of adult deaths: A validation study. Lancet. 2012 Jan 14;**379**(9811):136-142. DOI: 10.1016/S0140-6736(11)61483-9

[53] Goldman L, Sayson R, Robbins S, Cohn LH, Bettmann M, Weisberg M. The value of the autopsy in three medical eras. The New England Journal of Medicine. 1983 Apr 28;**308**(17):1000-1005

Chapter 3

Negative Autopsy in Infant and Juvenile Population: Role of Cardiac Arrhythmias

Georgia Sarquella-Brugada, Sergi Cesar,
Anna Fernandez-Falgueras,
Maria Dolores Zambrano, Anna Iglesias,
Josep Brugada, Ramon Brugada and
Oscar Campuzano

Additional information is available at the end of the chapter

http://dx.doi.org/10.5772/intechopen.71042

Abstract

Negative autopsy is a post-mortem examination in which a comprehensive analysis does not provide a cause of death. These include situation of death, anatomical and histological analysis, toxicology and microbiological study. A low part of autopsies remain without a conclusive cause of death, but all these cases are usually seen in young population, apparently healthy who died suddenly and unexpectedly. In these situations a cardiac arrhythmia is suspected as cause of death and genetic testing is recommended despite not regularly performed. Sudden death is a natural and unexpected decease that occurs in apparently healthy people, or whose disease was not severe enough to expect a fatal outcome. It can be due to several pathologies, usually of cardiac cause and called sudden cardiac death. In infants and young people, both long QT syndrome and catecholaminergic polymorphic ventricular tachycardia are main causes in negative autopsies. These genetic diseases lead to ventricular fibrillation, syncope and sudden cardiac death in a normal heart. Unfortunately, sudden cardiac death could be the first manifestation of the diseases, being early identification and prevention a crucial point in current medical practice. This chapter focuses on sudden death and negative autopsy in young population, mainly due to cardiac arrhythmias.

Keywords: sudden cardiac death, negative autopsy, arrhythmia, long QT syndrome, genetics

1. Introduction

An autopsy is a post-mortem examination of a deceased person in order to unravel the cause and time of death. In 5% of all cases, the autopsy may be classified as negative, concerning that no conclusive cause of death is identified after comprehensive analysis of all data recompiled. These data included gross and microscopically examination, and laboratory investigations [1]. Hence, unexplained death or "*mors sine materia*" is defined as "*the death that remains unsolved after a thorough autopsy, of an individual without previous cardiac history and who has been seen alive within the previous 12 hours of the death*" [2]. In these situations, cardiac death due to electric disorders without heart structural alterations could be considered the most common origin of the death [3]. Most part of these SD occurs in infants -sudden infant death syndrome (SIDS)-, and young population [4]. The two main disease associated with cardiac arrhythmias are long QT syndrome (LQTS) and catecholaminergic polymorphic ventricular tachycardia (CPVT). Both arrhythmias are of genetic origin and characterized with typical parameters in the electrocardiogram (ECG). For this reason, preventive medicine recommends to perform an ECG in all infants and young population (at least one ECG before 14 years old) in order to identify ECG alterations and, if positive, adopt preventive therapeutic measures to avoid a malignant arrhythmia. Unfortunately, the first manifestation of one cardiac arrhythmia may be the SCD, without previous symptoms.

Genetic analysis in post-mortem patients (also called molecular autopsy) may identify the genetic alteration responsible for an arrhythmogenic cardiac disease [5]. Current guidelines recommend performing the molecular autopsy in all these cases as a part of the comprehensive medico-legal investigation in SCD cases [6] but post-mortem genetic testing of the proband was reported in a low percentage of SCD cases with no structural alterations patients [7–9], mainly because forensic centers do not have the economic resources to perform genetic testing or do not collect samples due to currently legal restrictions involved with the sampling and storage of DNA [10]. Use of next generation sequencing technology (NGS) allows a comprehensive genetic analysis of all genes associated with SCD and cardiac arrhythmias, in a reduced time and in a cost-effective way, solving the economic problem. Due to genetic origin, family members could be also affected by the disease and at risk of SCD, despite asymptomatic. Therefore, both clinical and genetic analysis should be performed in all relatives, and interviewing family members may reveal helpful information not discovered in the initial research. It has been recommended that all relatives of unexplained SD victims undergo evaluation by a multidisciplinary team of cardiologists, forensic pathologists and geneticists [7] because of the investigation of an unexplained SD is extremely complicated in the families of the victims, mainly when the victim is a child (SIDS) [11, 12].

2. Inherited arrhythmias

Nowadays, nearly 85% of all SD are of cardiac origin (SCD) being responsible for around 30–200/100.000 yearly [13]. In population major 50 years old, around 80% of SCD cases are consequence of coronary disease [14], but in the younger population (less than 35 years) the cause is mainly due to inherited arrhythmias of genetic origin [15]. This last collection of diseases can be classified into two main groups [16]:

2.1. Cardiomyopathies

Arrhythmia is induced by structural abnormalities. These anatomical modifications are caused by alterations in genes encoding three types of proteins: sarcomeric which mainly cause hypertrophic cardiomyopathy (HCM); cytoskeletal, which mainly cause dilated cardiomyopathy (DCM), and desmosomal alterations, which mainly cause arrhythmogenic cardiomyopathy (ACM) [17]. These diseases imply a structural alteration of the heart, usually identified during an autopsy examination. In early stages of the disease, the alteration may be only identified using microscopic analysis but not at gross level. Curiously, both in SIDS and young people died suddenly, recent studies identified genetic alteration associated with any of these diseases but without any cardiac alteration, neither macroscopic nor microscopic. It could be explained because of the first structural alterations induced by the disease occurs at ultramicroscopic level (identified using only electronic microscopic). The electrical disturbance prior to malignant arrhythmia could be induced by these ultra-structural alterations. Hence, negative autopsy of infant and young population carrying alterations in genes encoding cardiomyopathies should not be discarding without a comprehensive analysis [18].

2.2. Channelopathies

Arrhythmogenic substrate is found in the electrical properties of the heart because genetic alterations occur in genes encoding for ion channels, their subunits or associated proteins playing a key role in the function of the channel. Ion channel diseases are not accompanied by structural cardiac defects and their first manifestation is a malignant arrhythmia or even SCD [19]. Cardiac channelopathies may be clinically identified only by the presence of some characteristic ECG abnormalities [20]. However, incomplete penetrance and variable expressivity in inherited arrhythmogenic disorders imply that the distinctive ECG patterns that characterize these disorders may be masked. When a SD occurs in a healthy young individual with no previous symptoms of any disease, arrhythmia is suspected as explanation of the disease but only identification of a genetic alteration may help us to identify the cause of the arrhythmia, and therefore, the cause of the death. Nowadays, hundreds of pathogenic variants have been identified in more than 40 genes, affecting sodium, potassium or calcium ion currents and depending on which ion channel is affected, different syndromes will be present [21]. Nevertheless, the same syndrome may show a certain degree of overlap if different types of channel can be affected. However, knowledge is not limited to the familial form, as it opens up new hypotheses as to how the gene interacts with the environment, drugs, and damaged muscle, and how arrhythmias arise in acquired or non-inherited forms [22]. This group includes LQTS, CPVT but also Brugada syndrome (BrS), and short QT syndrome (SQTS), among others [23]. In this chapter we will focus mainly in these diseases because of negative autopsy implies no cardiac abnormalities identified during post-mortem examination.

3. Long QT syndrome

This lethal entity is characterized for a prolongation of the QT interval (QTc>460 ms women and >450 ms men). The clinical presentation can be variable, ranging from asymptomatic patients to syncope and even SCD, mainly due to ventricular tachyarrhythmias (*torsade de pointes*) in the setting of a structurally normal heart. The spectrum of ECG abnormalities inducing electrical instability includes notched or biphasic T waves and T wave alternant. The prevalence is estimated in 1 of 2500 individuals [24, 25] being one of the leading causes of SCD among infants and young population. In recent years, massive ECG screening in young population has been performed with success of lowering rates of SD among infants and athletes [26]. In all patients, beta-blocker administration at high doses is highly recommended because it decreases the risk of SCD although do not provide full protection. The dose is adjusted according to the medical tolerance to these drugs (www.torsades.org). Implantable cardioverter-defibrillator (ICD) implantation is mandatory for those patients having had an aborted SCD and for those at risk of fatal arrhythmias [27]. LQTS can be acquired (associated with drugs and electrolyte imbalance such as hypokalemia, hypocalcaemia and hypomagnesaemia) or congenital (associated with pathogenic alterations in ion channels and/or associated proteins). Currently, more than 1000 genetic alterations have been identified in 20 genes (*AKAP9, ANK2, CACNA1C, CALM1, CALM2, CALM3, CAV3, KCNE1, KCNE2, KCNH2, KCNJ2, KCNJ5, KCNQ1, RYR2, SCN1B, SCN4B, SCN5A, SNTA1, TRDN* and *TRPM4*). All these genes together are responsible for 80–85% of all LQT cases [28] (**Figure 1**). Major genes associated with LQTS are *KCNQ1* –type 1- (30–35%), *KCNH2* –type 2- (25–30%) and *SCN5A* type 3- (5–10%) which are responsible for 65–75% of all LQTS cases [29]. A negative autopsy of a young case died suddenly (usually during exercise but also at rest) (**Figure 2**) could be caused by this arrhythmogenic entity.

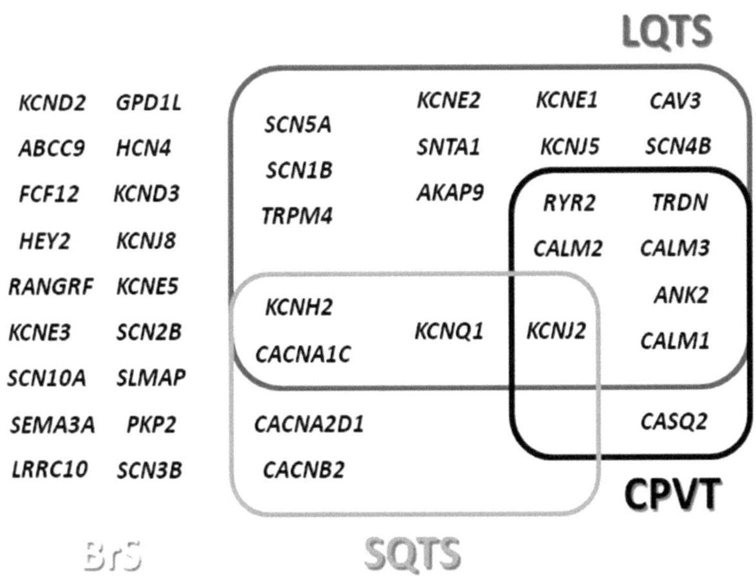

Figure 1. All genes associated with cardiac channelopathies. LQTS, long QT syndrome. BrS, Brugada syndrome. SQTS, short QT syndrome. CPVT, catecholaminergic polymorphic ventricular tachycardia.

http://dx.doi.org/10.5772/intechopen.71042

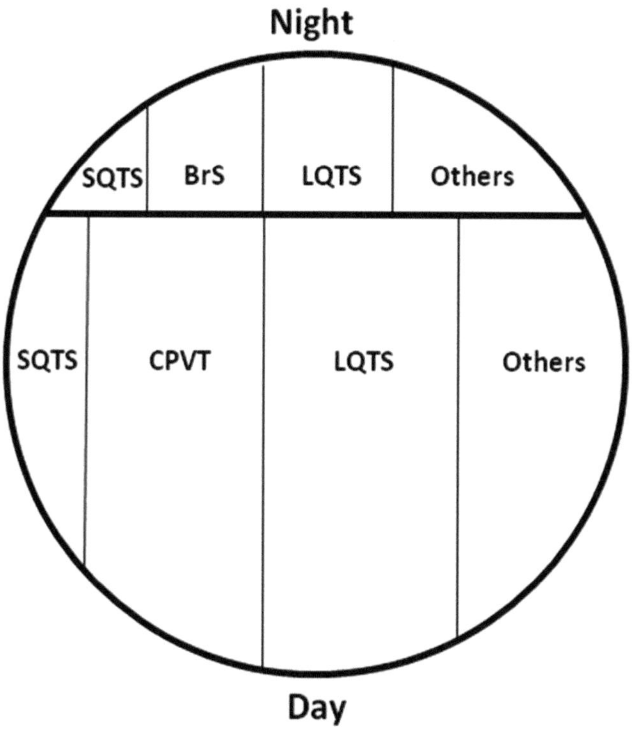

Figure 2. Distribution of arrhythmogenic diseases in negative autopsies. Most of deaths in young population before 16 years old occur during day. Adrenergic situations are the triggers of the arrhythmia during daily activities (exercise, emotion). The main diseases responsible for these sudden deaths are long QT syndrome (LQTS) and catecholaminergic polymorphic ventricular tachycardia (CPVT). A less proportion of deaths occur during night, meanly in infants before 2–3 years old. At rest, the main diseases associated with sudden death are LQTS and Brugada syndrome (BrS).

4. Catecholaminergic polymorphic ventricular tachycardia

This entity is an inherited disorder with a normal ECG at rest (occasionally with bradycardia, and U waves), and triggered exclusively by adrenergic stimulus (mainly exertion, extreme stress or emotion). It is characterized in the ECG by a 2-way polymorphic ventricular tachycardia in structural normal hearts [30]. It occurs mainly in children and adolescents and is increasingly recognized as a cause of unexplained SCD in young individuals, predominately in young males (30% by the age of 40 years) [31]. It was thought that the event happened in childhood (before age 10) with a high mortality rate [32]. Diagnosing CPVT can be difficult especially in young children. The first line of therapy is beta-blockers but ICDs are indicated for patients with aborted SCD or CPVT during exercise and in adolescents with incompletely controlled CPVT despite a high dose of medications [33]. Nowadays, more than 200 pathogenic alterations have been reported in 8 genes (*ANK2, CALM1, CALM2, CALM3, CASQ2, KCNJ2, RyR2* and *TRDN*) (**Figure 1**) and a comprehensive genetic analysis explains around 60% of CPVT cases. The main gene associated with CPVT is *RyR2*, being responsible of nearly 50% of all cases [34]. The ryanodine receptor is an intracellular calcium channel that is located in the sarcoplasmatic reticulum and activated by the influx of small amounts of calcium, thereby allowing the outflow of stored calcium, being crucial in triggering heart muscle contraction. A negative autopsy of a young case died suddenly during exercise could be caused by this arrhythmogenic entity (**Figure 2**).

5. Brugada syndrome

This inherited disease was identified in 1992 by Pedro and Josep Brugada [35]. It is characterized by an ECG pattern consisting of coved-type ST-segment elevation in atypical right-bundle branch block in leads V1 to V3 (often referred to as type-1 Brugada ECG pattern), and an increased risk for SCD resulting from episodes of polymorphic ventricular tachyarrhythmias. The ECG pattern can be baseline or intermittent, and it can be unmasked during a drug test (class IC sodium channel-blockers). The prevalence of the disease is 4–12% of all SCD causes. The penetrance and expressivity of the disorder are highly variable, although it is considered a disorder involving mainly young male adults (about 40 years old), and SCD typically occurring during sleep. Patients with BrS usually remain asymptomatic and modulating factors such as fever, exercise or drugs (www.brugadadrugs.org), may play a major role in the dynamic nature of the ECG. After surviving a cardiac arrest or the occurrence of syncope, the only treatment having any proven effect on the prevention of sudden death is the implantable cardioverter-defibrillator (ICD) [36]. However, ICD implantation in symptomatic is not free from controversy, especially in children [37]. The first genetic alteration was identified in 1998 [38]. Nowadays, 24 genes have been associated to the disease (*ABCC9, CACNA1C, CACNA2D1, CACNB2b, GPD1-L, HCN4, HEY2, KCND2, KCND3, KCNE3, KCNE5, KCNH2, KCNJ8, LRRC10, PKP2, RANGRF, SCN10A, SCN1B, SCN2B, SCN3B, SCN5A, SEMA3A, SLMAP* and *TRPM4*) (**Figure 1**) but a comprehensive genetic analysis only identify the genetic alteration in a 35% of cases. Approximately 30% of patients with BrS carry a loss of function genetic alteration in *SCN5A* (BrS type 1) [37]. This gene is responsible for the phase 0 of the cardiac action potential, a key player in the cardiac electrical activity. Hence, current guidelines only recommend genetic analysis of this gene [29]. A negative autopsy of a young case died during night could be caused by this arrhythmogenic entity (**Figure 2**).

6. Short QT syndrome

This arrhythmogenic disease was reported in 2000 [39]. It is a rare and highly lethal arrhythmic disease entity characterized by a short QT interval in ECG (<330 ms), with a high sharp T wave and a short interval between the peak and the end of the T wave, leading some clinical manifestations from lack of symptoms to syncope, and even SCD. Clinical manifestations may appear in infants and young population, being considered one of the main causes SIDS [40]. Nowadays there is no pharmacological therapy of proven efficacy to prevent arrhythmias and the implant of an ICD is the only alternative for high-risk cases. Nowadays, few pathogenic alterations have been identified in 6 different genes encoding potassium and calcium ion channels (*KCNQ1, KCNJ2, KCNH2, CACNA1C, CACNB2* and *CACNA2D1*)

(**Figure 1**), following an autosomal dominant pattern of inheritance [41]. It should be a high penetrance and a comprehensive genetic analysis identifies the genetic alteration in nearly 60% of clinically diagnosed cases. A negative autopsy of an infant case (less than 2 years) died suddenly could be caused by this arrhythmogenic entity (**Figure 2**).

7. Next generation sequencing

The genetic revolution was initiated 20 years ago, firstly with the knowledge of the human genome and in last 10 years with the advances in genetic technology that have permitted the development of massively parallel sequencing (also called next generation sequencing). Hence, current NGS technologies allow a massive sequencing of genes, even whole exome and genomes. The advance is the reduced time and the cost-effective way in comparison to traditional Sanger sequencing. Traditional Sanger sequencing has high fidelity but is slow and quite expensive compared with next generation methods. However, Sanger remains as a gold standard in validation of alterations as well as family segregation. In recent 5 years, NGS technology has been implemented in forensic area, allowing a comprehensive post-mortem genetic analysis. Hence, molecular autopsy using NGS has identified the cause of the death in a large part of cases with a no conclusive cause of death after comprehensive autopsy protocol without genetic analysis [42]. Current guidelines recommend use of molecular autopsy in young cases classified as negative after an autopsy [29]. The NGS analysis requires a certain DNA quality and quantity; the best approach is obtaining DNA from post-mortem blood, conserved at 4°C. DNA from tissue can be also an option but the conservation should be at −20°C. Currently, DNA from formalin-fixed, paraffin-embedded (FFPE) is not an option due to formalin destroy DNA and no proper amplification is possible for NGS technology. After NGS analysis, the next challenge is the interpretation of data identified. Most part of alterations remains as ambiguous significance and an exhaustive analysis of each variant should be performed before translation into clinical practice [43–45]. This will require sustained collaboration between geneticist, cardiologist and forensics for genetic data interpretation, to optimize cause of death in a negative autopsy but also in family members in order to adopt personalized therapies.

8. Conclusions

In infant and young population, unexpected SD remains as a main problem because usually the first manifestation of the disease is the death. In last 10 years, negative autopsy cases are being progressively more studied in order to identify the cause of death, especially in young population. Cases usually classified without conclusive cause of death have been comprehensively analyzed and resolved. However, molecular autopsy is not performed in all forensic centers and large percentage of cases remains without a cause of death. Use of genetics in forensic area has improved diagnosis of negative autopsies, but also identification of relatives at risk of SCD. Early identification of individuals at risk allows adoption of therapeutic measures in prevention of new lethal episodes in infant and young population.

Acknowledgements/funding

This work was supported by Fundació La Marató TV3 (358/U/2015), Obra Social 'La Caixa', Fundació Daniel Bravo and Fondo Investigacion Sanitaria (FIS PI14/01773) from the Instituto de Salud Carlos III (ISCIII). The CIBERCV is an initiative of the ISCIII, Spanish Ministry of Economy and Competitiveness.

Author details

Georgia Sarquella-Brugada[1], Sergi Cesar[1], Anna Fernandez-Falgueras[2], Maria Dolores Zambrano[1], Anna Iglesias[2,4], Josep Brugada[1,3,4], Ramon Brugada[2,4,5,6] and Oscar Campuzano[2,4,5]*

*Address all correspondence to: oscar@brugada.org

1 Arrhythmia Unit, Hospital Sant Joan de Déu, Barcelona, Spain

2 Cardiovascular Genetics Center, University of Girona-IDIBGI, Girona, Spain

3 Cardiovascular Institute, Hospital Clinic, University of Barcelona, Barcelona, Spain

4 Centro de Investigación Biomédica en Red de Enfermedades Cardiovasculares (CIBERCV), Spain

5 Medical Science Department, School of Medicine, University of Girona, Girona, Spain

6 Cardiology Service, Hospital Josep Trueta, Girona, Spain

References

[1] Lawler W. The negative coroner's necropsy: A personal approach and consideration of difficulties. Journal of Clinical Pathology. 1990;**43**:977-980

[2] Basso C, Burke M, Fornes P, et al. Guidelines for autopsy investigation of sudden cardiac death. Virchows Archiv. 2008;**452**:11-18

[3] Oliva A, Brugada R, D'Aloja E, et al. State of the art in forensic investigation of sudden cardiac death. The American Journal of Forensic Medicine and Pathology. 2011;Mar;**32**(1):1-16

[4] Tfelt-Hansen J, Winkel BG, Grunnet M, Jespersen T. Cardiac channelopathies and sudden infant death syndrome. Cardiology. 2011;**119**:21-33

[5] Campuzano O, Sanchez-Molero O, Allegue C, et al. Post-mortem genetic analysis in juvenile cases of sudden cardiac death. Forensic Science International. 2014;**245C**:30-37

[6] Wedekind H, Schulze-Bahr E, Debus V, et al. Cardiac arrhythmias and sudden death in infancy: Implication for the medicolegal investigation. International Journal of Legal Medicine. 2007;**121**:245-257

[7] Behr E, Wood DA, Wright M, et al. Cardiological assessment of first-degree relatives in sudden arrhythmic death syndrome. Lancet. 2003;**362**:1457-1459

[8] Tan HL, Hofman N, van Langen IM, et al. Sudden unexplained death: Heritability and diagnostic yield of cardiological and genetic examination in surviving relatives. Circulation. 2005;**112**:207-213

[9] Behr ER, Dalageorgou C, Christiansen M, et al. Sudden arrhythmic death syndrome: Familial evaluation identifies inheritable heart disease in the majority of families. European Heart Journal. 2008;**29**:1670-1680

[10] Michaud K, Mangin P, Elger BS. Genetic analysis of sudden cardiac death victims: A survey of current forensic autopsy practices. International Journal of Legal Medicine. 2011;**125**:359-366

[11] Klaver EC, Versluijs GM, Wilders R. Cardiac ion channel mutations in the sudden infant death syndrome. International Journal of Cardiology. 2011;**152**:162-170

[12] Dettmeyer RB, Kandolf R. Cardiomyopathies—Misdiagnosed as Sudden Infant Death Syndrome (SIDS). Forensic Science International. 2010;**194**(1-3):e21-e24. doi: 10.1016/j.forsciint.2009.10.010

[13] Podrid PJ, Myerburg RJ. Epidemiology and stratification of risk for sudden cardiac death. Clinical Cardiology. 2005;**28**:I3-I11

[14] Myerburg RJ, Junttila MJ. Sudden cardiac death caused by coronary heart disease. Circulation. 2012;**125**:1043-1052

[15] Arzamendi D, Benito B, Tizon-Marcos H, et al. Increase in sudden death from coronary artery disease in young adults. American Heart Journal. 2011;**161**:574-580

[16] Deo R, Albert CM. Epidemiology and genetics of sudden cardiac death. Circulation. 2012;**125**:620-637

[17] Oliva A, Grassi VM, Campuzano O, et al. Medico-legal perspectives on sudden cardiac death in young athletes. International Journal of Legal Medicine. 2017;**131**:393-409

[18] Sarquella-Brugada G, Campuzano O, Cesar S, et al. Sudden infant death syndrome caused by cardiac arrhythmias: Only a matter of genes encoding ion channels? International Journal of Legal Medicine. 2016;**130**:415-420

[19] Fernández-Falgueras A, Sarquella-Brugada G, Brugada J, et al. Cardiac channelopathies and sudden death: Recent clinical and genetic advances. Biology (Basel). 2017 Jan 29;**6**(1). pii: E7. doi: 10.3390/biology6010007. Review. PMID: 28146053

[20] Schimpf R, Veltmann C, Wolpert C, Borggrefe M. Channelopathies: Brugada syndrome, long QT syndrome, short QT syndrome, and CPVT. Herz. 2009;**34**:281-288

[21] Campuzano O, Sarquella-Brugada G, Brugada R, Brugada J. Genetics of channelopathies associated with sudden cardiac death. Global Cardiology Science & Practice. 2015;**2015**:39

[22] Roberts R. The number one cause for sudden cardiac death in the young unravels. Cardiology. 2010;**115**:46-48

[23] Campuzano O, Allegue C, Partemi S, et al. Negative autopsy and sudden cardiac death. International Journal of Legal Medicine. 2014;**128**:599-606

[24] Lupoglazoff JM, Denjoy I, Guicheney P, et al. Congenital long QT syndrome. Archives de Pédiatrie. 2001;**8**:525-534

[25] Moss AJ, Shimizu W, Wilde AA, et al. Clinical aspects of type-1 long-QT syndrome by location, coding type, and biophysical function of mutations involving the KCNQ1 gene. Circulation. 2007;**115**:2481-2489

[26] Mizusawa Y, Horie M, Wilde AA. Genetic and clinical advances in congenital long QT syndrome. Circulation Journal. 2014;**78**:2827-2833

[27] Behere SP, Shubkin CD, Weindling SN. Recent advances in the understanding and management of long QT syndrome. Current Opinion in Pediatrics. 2014;**26**:727-733

[28] Nakano Y, Shimizu W. Genetics of long-QT syndrome. Journal of Human Genetics. 2016;**61**:51-55

[29] Priori SG, Blomstrom-Lundqvist C. 2015 European Society of Cardiology Guidelines for the management of patients with ventricular arrhythmias and the prevention of sudden cardiac death summarized by co-chairs. European Heart Journal. 2015;**36**:2757-2759

[30] Refaat MM, Hassanieh S, Scheinman M. Catecholaminergic polymorphic ventricular tachycardia. Cardiac Electrophysiology Clinics. 2016;**8**:233-237

[31] Mohamed U, Napolitano C, Priori SG. Molecular and electrophysiological bases of catecholaminergic polymorphic ventricular tachycardia. Journal of Cardiovascular Electrophysiology. 2007;**18**:791-797

[32] Ylanen K, Poutanen T, Hiippala A, et al. Catecholaminergic polymorphic ventricular tachycardia. European Journal of Pediatrics. 2010;**169**:535-542

[33] Imberti JF, Underwood K, Mazzanti A, Priori SG. Clinical challenges in catecholaminergic polymorphic ventricular tachycardia. Heart, Lung & Circulation. 2016;Aug;**25**(8):777-783

[34] Laitinen PJ, Brown KM, Piippo K, et al. Mutations of the cardiac ryanodine receptor (RyR2) gene in familial polymorphic ventricular tachycardia. Circulation. 2001;**103**:485-490

[35] Brugada P, Brugada J. Right bundle branch block, persistent ST segment elevation and sudden cardiac death: A distinct clinical and electrocardiographic syndrome. A multi-center report. Journal of the American College of Cardiology. 1992;**20**:1391-1396

[36] Benito B, Brugada R, Brugada J, Brugada P. Brugada syndrome. Progress in Cardiovascular Diseases. 2008;**51**:1-22

[37] Sarquella-Brugada G, Campuzano O, Arbelo E, et al. Brugada syndrome: Clinical and genetic findings. Genetics in Medicine. 2016;**18**:3-12

[38] Brugada P, Benito B, Brugada R, Brugada J. Brugada syndrome: Update 2009. Hellenic Journal of Cardiology. 2009;**50**:352-372

[39] Gussak I, Brugada P, Brugada J, et al. Idiopathic short QT interval: A new clinical syndrome? Cardiology. 2000;**94**:99-102

[40] Pereira R, Campuzano O, Sarquella-Brugada G, et al. Short QT syndrome in pediatrics. Clinical Research in Cardiology. 2017; Jun;**106**(6):393-400

[41] Behere SP, Weindling SN. Inherited arrhythmias: The cardiac channelopathies. Annals of Pediatric Cardiology. 2015;**8**:210-220

[42] Sanchez O, Campuzano O, Fernandez-Falgueras A, et al. Natural and undetermined sudden death: Value of post-mortem genetic investigation. PLoS One. 2016;**11**:e0167358

[43] Campuzano O, Allegue C, Fernandez A, et al. Determining the pathogenicity of genetic variants associated with cardiac channelopathies. Scientific Reports. 2015;**5**:7953

[44] Richards S, Aziz N, Bale S, et al. Standards and guidelines for the interpretation of sequence variants: A joint consensus recommendation of the American College of Medical Genetics and Genomics and the Association for Molecular Pathology. Genetics in Medicine. 2015;**17**:405-424

[45] Amendola LM, Jarvik GP, Leo MC, et al. Performance of ACMG-AMP variant-interpretation guidelines among nine laboratories in the Clinical Sequencing Exploratory Research consortium. American Journal of Human Genetics. 2016;**98**:1067-1076

Chapter 4

Postmortem Animal Attacks on Human Corpses

Zerrin Erkol and Erdem Hösükler

Additional information is available at the end of the chapter

http://dx.doi.org/10.5772/intechopen.72929

Abstract

Postmortem animal activity is an important step in incorporating protein, fat, and carbohydrates in corpses to the food chain. Many animal species are members of this food chain. Outdoor corpses may be attacked by many predacious and scavenger animals and exposed to complete destruction, and bones and belongings of the dead person may be scattered all over a large area due to postmortem animal activity. Indoor corpses may be attacked by pets, domestic dogs, cats, ants, and rodents during postmortem period. Besides, if the corpse is in shallow water, other terrestrial predators may harm the corpse. The most important issue in the presence of lesions on the corpse caused by animals is to accurately discriminate between antemortem and postmortem wounds. The extent of the lesions caused by the animals varies according to the sizes of their dentition and jaws, but they share some common characteristics. Lack of bleeding from bitten tissue excepting small amount of extravasated blood, absence of active bleeding, edema, and erythema on the edges of the wound are among these shared characteristics. In this chapter, the subject of postmortem animal attacks on human corpses will be evaluated by revising the recent references.

Keywords: forensic sciences, crime scene investigation, decomposition, postmortem animal attacks, postmortem animal injury, animal scavengers, carnivores, postmortem artifacts, teeth marks, dispersed remains

1. Introduction

1.1. Postmortem animal scavenging activity, motivation, pattern and forensic problems

Animal activity on corpses during postmortem period plays an important role in the integration of protein, fat, and carbohydrate contents of the corpse into the food chain and constitutes an important part of the taphonomic process experienced by the body after death [1, 2]. Many animal species are members of this food chain. In order to identify the animal that attacked the corpse, the location of the corpse, geographic conditions, season, animal species found in the area, types of animal feeding, and behaviors should be known [3]. Indoor corpses may be attacked by many predacious and scavenger animals and exposed to complete destruction, and bones and belongings of the dead person may be scattered all over a large area due to postmortem animal activity [4, 5]. Outdoor corpses may be attacked by pets, domestic dogs, cats, ants, and rodents during postmortem period [6–13]. If the corpse was immersed in water, then many aquatic animals as fish, water rats, crabs, and amphipods may attack the corpse [14–16]. Besides, if the corpse is in shallow water, other terrestrial predators may harm the corpse [1].

Devouring the remains of human corpses by animals may cause many problems concerning forensic pathology and forensic anthropology:

1. If serious destructive changes occur especially on the face of the corpse and teeth, then identification of the corpse may be difficult [6, 7, 9–12, 17].
2. Even if the individual died because of natural consequences, when the internal organs are devoured by animals, then it might be impossible to identify the precise cause of death [17–19].
3. During postmortem period, lesions caused by animal attacks may be evaluated and misinterpreted as antemortem lesions as ligature mark, firearm wound, or stab wound [2, 7, 9, 10, 13, 20].
4. At the time of dying, clothes may be opened, and exposed genital organs may be depredated by animals during postmortem period, which may raise the suspicion of sexual mutilation [17, 21].
5. In posttraumatic deaths, open wounds may be the first target of scavengers, and within a very short time, precise identification of antemortem wounds may become seriously complicated [22, 23].
6. During postmortem period, existence of living beings such as ants, which feed on both the corpse, and adult and larvae of flies and insects, putrefaction of the corpse may be delayed because of devouring of eggs, and larvae. Faunal succession of insects and flies, which is especially used to determine the postmortem interval, may change leading to erroneous estimation of the postmortem interval [4, 24].
7. Loss of skin may lead to disappearance of tattoos and old surgical scars, which may be used for identification of the victim [18].

Hunger is the main factor for animal motivation in outdoor postmortem animal scavenging. The odors pervading from the corpse due to natural putrefaction process attract the attention of wild animals [25]. This condition differs slightly for domestic animals. Domestic animals frequently do not feel the need to hunt for nutrition. It has been indicated that for postmortem scavenging activity of domestic cats and dogs living in confined spaces, the corpse should belong to a socially isolated individual living alone at home and also there should be a pet (cats and dogs) moving freely at home, but cannot reach its food [26]. In contrast, dogs feeding on their owner's corpse during postmortem period as reported in some cases cited in the literature cannot be solely explained by only starvation. Rothschild and Schneider [27] presented a case of a 31-year-old male who was living with his mother and an Alsatian dog. The victim had postmortem scavenging wounds on his face and neck formed by his dog after he had committed suicide with a firearm. Interestingly, only 45 minutes had elapsed from the time the man shot himself to the head and the discovery of the corpse. This time interval was not considered to be long enough for the dog to become hungry. Besides, near the bed of the victim's corpse, a half-filled canned food and a bowl full of dog food were found. According to Rothschild and Schneider [27], the most probable explanation of this condition was that the pet began to lick and poke its unconscious owner with the intention to help him. However, when its attempts failed, the authors claimed that the dog had become more aggressive and had bitten its owner so as to arouse him, and they defined this as displacement behavior. In a case presentation, a man died due to a coronary problem was wounded by his hunting dog only a few hours after his death, which according to authors' opinions could not be explained by hunger of the dog or deficient food [28]. Buschman et al. [12] presented three cases that had been attacked by pet dogs during postmortem period, and they reported that dog foods were accessible in all these three events. Rossi et al. [29] presented a case in which the victim's nose and mouth were injured by her dog during postmortem period. Witnesses said that they had seen the victim had drunk a lot and had become unconscious when she was alive, and her red setter dog had bitten her legs and licked her face to arouse her. If the animal is locked for a long time, as a "displacement" behavior, its postmortem scavenging activity starts from the face of the victim and proceeds toward the lower part of the body, and finally, the abdomen is devoured [30]. In other words, initially, scavenging activity starts as a "displacement" behavior, and then as a result of the animal confined in a closed space, it continues as a result of starvation. Besides longer periods of confinement may induce aggressive behaviors in dogs, which may contribute to postmortem mutilation [11]. Furthermore, concerning human being–dog hierarchy, in case of weakness of its owner, dominancy may change in favor of the dog. In this case, a type of "mental disease" develops in the dog, and the dog may feel itself compelled to attack its owner and display aggressive behaviors against him/her to prove its leadership [25, 27, 29, 31, 32].

If postmortem feeding is prolonged, then the scavenger may have left teeth marks on the victim's bones. Basically, bite marks caused by predatory animals include pits, punctures, scores, and furrows [33]. Pits are caused by collapsing of the bone under masticatory forces created by the tip of the teeth during chewing act, but they do not penetrate into the bone cortex [34–37]. Punctures are formed by greater force exerted by teeth on bone with resultant penetration of the tip of the teeth into cortical bone. Frequently, it is seen in thin and flat bones as scapula, and it is caused by canine and carnassial teeth [21, 34, 37]. A score is a bite mark longer than three times its width. It is formed by dragging or rotatory movement of the tooth on the bone after formation of a pit [5, 21, 34, 38]. Scorings are scratches extending parallel to the long axis of the bone, which are seen as "V" or cube-shaped marks on cross section of the bone [23]. Furrows are deeply formed channel-like grooves that extend longitudinally along the long bones as femur and formed by molar and premolar teeth of the animals that repeat jaw movements with the intention to reach the bone marrow [21, 25, 33, 34]. However, if a scavenger spends lots of time in chewing, then it creates furrows and pits on the bone, which makes it impossible to discern individual teeth marks due to its continuous mumbling of the bone between its upper and lower jaws [6, 21, 25].

When the outdoor corpses are left out for a sufficient period of time, then scavengers may devour the corpse leaving only bones [33, 39, 40]. In such cases, analysis and interpretation of defective skeletal remains are requested from forensic anthropologist [19, 34, 40, 41]. Indeed, during or after feeding, these animals may change the anatomical location of bones. However, studies performed have indicated that scavenging behavior and pattern of these animals are not usually coincidental [4, 5, 25, 42–44]. Haglund et al. [41] investigated destructive changes induced by jackals and pet dogs on partially or completely skeletonized remains of human corpses created within a period ranging between 4 hours and 52 months so as to search for scavenging activity. As a result, they defined stages of disarticulation secondary to scavenging behaviors of jackals and dogs. Accordingly, the following disarticulation sequence was defined: Stage 0: No evidence of disarticulation and loss of soft tissues at an early phase (postmortem 4 hours–14 days); Stage 1: Fragmentized ventral thorax characterized by loss of sternum, destruction of sternal ribs, evisceration, loss of scapula, partial/total loss of clavicula, and loss of one or both upper extremities (postmortem 22 days–2.5 months); Stage 2: In addition to stage 1, it also involves the lower extremities (postmortem 2–4.5 months); Stage 3: All parts of the skeleton excluding the vertebra are fragmentized, seriously injured, and destroyed. During this stage, bones are scattered at a distance varying between 3 and 91 m (postmortem 2–11 months); Stage 4: Total disarticulation (postmortem 6–52 months). However, some disarticulation patterns do not fit into these categories (18). Indeed, only three cases of four postmortem attacks by pet animals presented by Rossi et al. [29] are in concordance with disarticulation sequence defined by Haglund, while in the third case, where the culprit was a German shepherd dog, face, neck, intrathoracic organs, upper right extremity, scapula, and multiple number of cervical and thoracic vertebrae of the victim had been reportedly devoured.

The most important issue in the presence of lesions on the corpse caused by animals is to accurately discriminate between antemortem and postmortem wounds. In postmortem injuries, any defense wound on the victim's corpse is not present [26, 45, 46]. However, absence of defense wound on the deceased does not always signify wounds created during postmortem period. Salem et al. [47] presented a 27-year-old epileptic woman found dead at her home. Wide lesions on the neck of the corpse created by the domestic mongrel dog were found without any defense wounds on her body. However, on histological analysis of the wound, specimen hemorrhagic reactions were found in cutaneous, subcutaneous, and muscle tissue, which are signs of vitality. The authors asserted that the dog attacked the victim during an epileptic attack when she had lost her consciousness. Only a little amount of blood extravasated passively from the vessels of the tissue of the wound created during postmortem period [7, 9, 12, 19, 21, 48]. Besides, edema and redness on the edges of the wound that are signs of vitality are not observed [2, 21, 31, 49, 50]. Numerous histological, histochemical, and immunohistochemical methods can be used to determine whether animal attack occurred during antemortem or postmortem period. Cell types functioning in wound healing and changes in the wound with time may be determined using histological examination [51]. During histochemical examination, fibroblastic enzymes (esterases, acid phosphatase, and ATPase) may be analyzed. However, these tests have a lower reliability [52]. It has been indicated that in immunohistochemical analysis adhesion molecules as P-selectin, E-selectin, ICAM-1, VCAM-1 [53–55], inflammatory cytokines as fibronectin [56], IL-1, IL-6, TNF [57], and transforming growth factor (TGF) [58] can be used to discriminate between antemortem and postmortem wounds. Hernández-Cueto et al. [59] indicated that levels of D-dimer are significantly higher in antemortem skin wounds relative to postmortem wounds. Ortiz-Rey et al. [60] reported that fibronectin and tenascin increase in most of the antemortem wounds. They indicated that still it was not a specific finding and yielded positive results in association with passive extravasation of these molecules from damaged blood vessels in postmortem wounds. He and Zhu [61] investigated 13 antemortem and 7 postmortem skin lesions of 7 forensic cases and determined that leukotriene B4 (LTB4) was found in all antemortem wound samples, while it was not detected in any one of the postmortem wound samples.

1.2. Attacks of land animals during postmortem period

Consequences of postmortem animal attacks at the corpse on land differ depending on whether the corpse is in outdoor or indoor environment. Outdoor corpses may be devoured by many animals because they are defenseless. Flies and worms are most prevalently associated with decomposition of the body [2, 17, 62]. Adult insects leave their eggs on moist regions of the body, namely on wounds, eyes, lips, and genital region of fresh corpses, and with time, many herds of larvae of specific species come out of the eggs and develop [1]. Larvae may cover the corpse completely, erase potentially diagnostic cutaneous marks such as tattoos and surgical scars, and damage internal organs making determination of precise cause of death impossible [17]. Worms release proteolytic digestive secretions and thus soften tissues and create subcutaneous tunnels and sinuses during their passage, which accelerate putrefaction of the corpse [1]. These holes opened by worms may sometimes resemble wounds created by bullets [2, 63]. Although rare, enzymes secreted from salivary glands of fly larvae may puncture bone lamellae (i.e., orbital ceiling) [63]. However larvae may cause skin defects, which may be confused with penetrating stab wounds formed by sharp objects [1, 17, 49]. Moreover, some authors have claimed that swelling only due to decomposition and decay incurred by worms may disarray clothes, which can be seen as attempts of sexual assault [64]. Via evaluating developmental stages of insects and insect genome sequences on the corpse, postmortem interval can be determined [65–70]. Besides, in severely decayed corpses, DNA of the deceased can be identified by analyzing gastrointestinal contents of worms feeding on the corpse [71, 72].

Ants, which are among one of the dominant insect groups, belong to *Formicidae* family of *Hymenoptera spp.* [24]. Ants feed on outdoor copses, but they may damage indoor copses such as in homes and garden cottages [8]. Typically, ants start to appear a short time after death, and they may also be seen on the corpse or in its close vicinity during advanced decomposition phases of the corpse. Ants feed on adult flies and insects and their larvae, flesh, and exudates of the corpse, and they may decrease the decomposition rate significantly [24]. Ants also form colonies of queen, soldier, and worker ants and may become the dominant arthropods on the corpse. Goff and Win [73] estimated postmortem interval of a corpse based on minimum colony forming period of *Anoplolepis Longipes* (*Hymenoptera*: *Formicidae*) species of ants as 12 months. Postmortem ant feeding causes formation of generally superficial, serpiginous, parchmentized, and irregular-shaped skin lesions [8, 17, 24] (**Figure 1**). Besides, small punctate and scratch-type lesions that can be confused with antemortem abrasion and acid wounds may be seen [24]. Injuries caused by ants generally leave behind orange-pink wound marks scattered on the skin surface [24]. Ants usually feed on exposed areas of the body and

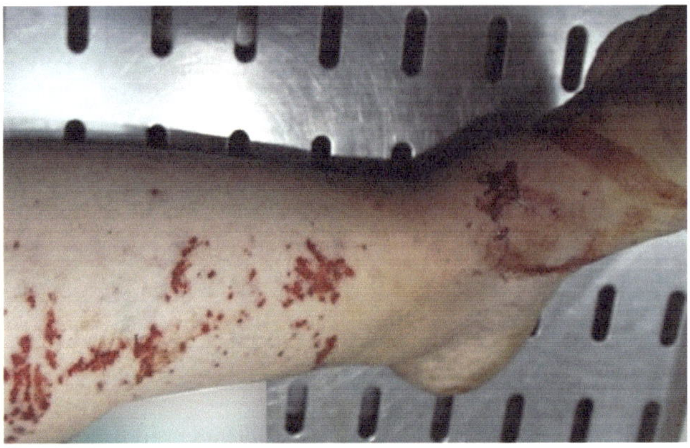

Figure 1. Serpiginous, parchmentized, and irregular-shaped superficial skin lesions were associated with postmortem ant activity on the left leg (Archive of Council of Forensic Medicine, Turkey).

edges of the clothes. Most frequently, the areas they prefer are lips, eyelids, and joints [1]. However, it has been asserted that removal of eyelashes is the characteristic activity of ants [17]. Ant bites remove the most upper layer of the skin and dermis, and underlying structures are exposed. In other words, ant bites generally cause lesions characterized by absence of only epidermal layer. This skin damage does not lead to bleeding excepting passive oozing of the blood from the ends of traumatized dermal capillaries [8]. When lesions associated with post-mortem ant activity are localized on the neck, it might be erroneously interpreted as hanging marks [1, 2, 17, 24]. Besides, from regions of congestion developed because of remaining of the corpse at the same position for a long term, terminal ends of dermal capillaries bitten by ants may seriously bleed, which may be misinterpreted by investigators as signs of trauma [8, 17]. Byard presented a case of a 59-year-old victim whose autopsy revealed ischemic heart disease as the cause of death. At the incident site, lesions at the right side of the victim's forehead due to ant bites, ants moving on his face, and blood around his head had been reported [17]. Byard [8] detected congested face due to hanging, widespread lesions around neck and chin caused by ant bites, and diffuse blood spots on the face and shirt of a 51-year-old hanging victim. These cases demonstrate that recording the presence of ants especially at incident site will facilitate the work of the physician who will perform the autopsy.

Postmortem wounds caused by cockroaches are typically seen on extremities covered by tunnel-like clothing. Cockroaches may cause superficial dermal abrasions resembling skin diseases [2].

Predators as rodents also devour tissues of the dead body most dramatically as insects [13, 48]. Rodents (mouse, rat, hamster, etc.) have a total of 16 teeth, including 2 incisors and 6 molar teeth both in the upper and lower jaws [74] (**Figure 2**). Parallel cutaneous lesions and fine serrated wound contours on corpses caused by upper and lower incisor teeth of the rodents during postmortem feeding are observed [9, 10, 13, 48, 74] (**Figures 3** and **4**). Irregular edges of wounds due to repetitive gnawing may be seen [10]. If the bone is also gnawed, then parallel scratches or furrows may be formed at the edges of the bone [13, 25, 37]. Rodents may feed on corpses both in the open air and in confined space as home [9, 13, 25, 37, 48, 74]. Rodent

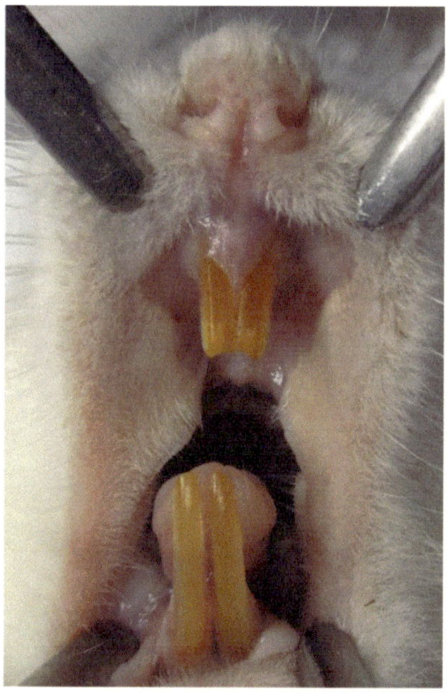

Figure 2. Two incisor teeth both in the upper and lower jaws in a rat.

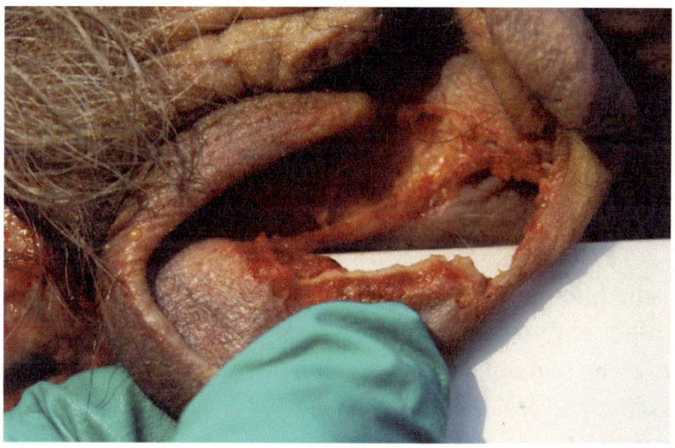

Figure 3. Soft and cartilaginous tissue loss due to postmortem rodent activity in right ear and irregular serrated appearance at wound edge (Archive of Council of Forensic Medicine, Turkey).

activity has been reported more frequently in lower socioeconomic living conditions and among homeless people [26]. At the incident site, the presence of rodent feces should suggest postmortem rodent activity [9, 13]. Especially when indoor postmortem rodent interference is suspected, searching for rodent nest at the incident site facilitates establishment of accurate diagnosis [13, 74]. Ropohl et al. [74] presented a case of a 43-year-old woman whose hip and lower abdominal and genital regions were naked, which raised the suspicion of a sexual assault. At the incident site, widespread tissue defects on the face of the victim and rodent feces and in a drawer a golden hamster wrapped in paper towels were found. In the nest of

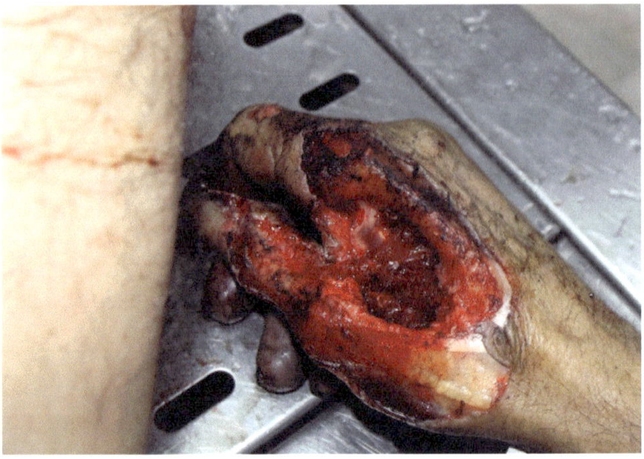

Figure 4. Soft tissue defect of the right hand due to postmortem rodent activity. Irregular wound margin and disclosed underlying muscle and tendon (Archive of Council of Forensic Medicine, Turkey).

the hamster made up of these paper towels, pea-shaped tissue and muscle fragments were detected. When the rodent has enough time for feeding, it devours naked, unclothed, easily accessible parts of the body such as face and arms, till bones, (**Figure 5**) and this situation may create problems in identification of the victim. In the author's own case, a 75–80-year-old solitary woman in bad socioeconomic status was found dead at home. Widespread soft tissue and muscle loss on face, neck, and upper extremities that exposed the underlying bone tissue were observed. Both of her hands were amputated from the wrists. On the edges of the wounds, teeth marks peculiar to rats were detected, and pneumonia was implicated for her cause of death [75] (**Figure 6a, b**).

Rodents may harm the corpse within a very short time. A 41-year-old homeless victim was found dead inside an arbor. It was determined that postmortem rodent injuries, detected at autopsy but not in the photographs taken at the scene and in the reports of the scene investigator, had taken place within a short time as approximately 45–60 minutes [13]. Byard [17] reported two victims who had bullet entry holes on the nasal root, which deformed with postmortem rodent activity, and lesions on hands caused by rodent activity had been confused with defense wounds.

Vultures, eagles, ravens, magpies, and many species of birds can feed on corpses [4, 5, 39, 62, 76, 77]. Birds primarily tend to feed on eyes of the corpses. This condition may lead to misinterpretations by crime scene investigators as a sadistically committed crime or ritual mutilation performed on the corpse [17]. Scavenger birds as magpies and crows peck and tear the corpse during feeding, which causes characteristic triangle-shaped holes on the corpse [76]. Dettling et al. [78] demonstrated unusual patched areas of epidermal lesions on naked unclothed parts of a dead woman caused by scavenging activity of songbird characterized by "pecking and dragging." In another case, loss of eye globe and earlobe due to crow feeding was reported [79]. Variations in beak morphologies of birds may cause different lesions. Vultures and falcons may leave wounds with smooth contours resembling surgical cuts after plucking the skin [76]. Birds can tear away intact skin, but they primarily prefer to feed on

http://dx.doi.org/10.5772/intechopen.72929

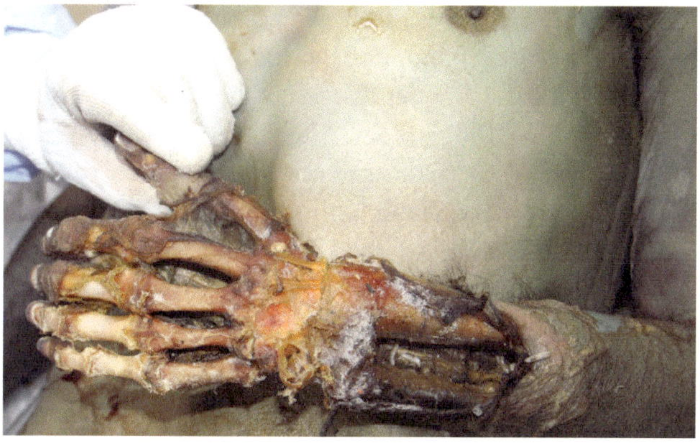

Figure 5. Widespread muscle and soft tissue loss disclosed skeletal tissue due to long-term postmortem rodent activity (Archive of Council of Forensic Medicine, Turkey).

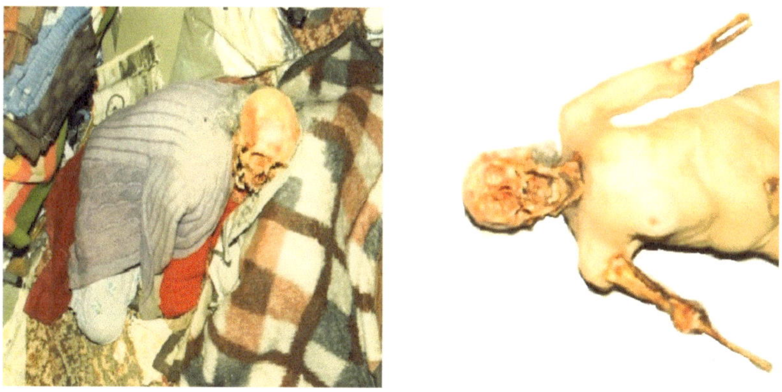

Figure 6. The incident site of the corpse of a 75–80-year-old woman who was living alone in low socioeconomic level is shown in (a). Amputated hand, extensive soft tissue, and muscle loss that exposed bone tissue of head, neck, and upper extremity caused by postmortem activity of rodents are seen in (b).

the places where skin integrity is disrupted or eroded. If the corpse is exposed to penetrating trauma during perimortem period, then birds frequently focus on this injured region, and a large round hole may occur due to feeding [76]. In a study on the most known scavenger bird, namely vultures, it was reported that vultures observe the corpse for 24 hours before feeding on it, and during 4–5 hours of active feeding period, they can skeletonize the corpse [80]. Conversely, in an observational study, Beck et al. [5] left pig carcasses in an open field and indicated that vultures had started to feed on the corpse 17 days later, which they attributed to raining that suppressed the spread of odor of the carcass. In addition, some studies with 37 days of follow-up period have been also cited [39]. If crows and magpies want to feed on larvae in cancellous bone, they will remove outer cortical layer of the bone and cause cone-shaped lesions in the cancellous bone. These cone-shaped lesions caused by beaks of the birds do not demonstrate any symmetry. These lesions are haphazardly placed, and frequently they overlap. Destructive changes seem to focus on a certain area. Birds focus on an area of soft tissue to create a round hole, and also they target a certain part of the bone, remove the cortical layer, and create a collapsed area on the cancellous bone. Birds frequently leave their teeth marks on the center of the long bones or flat parts of irregularly shaped bones as scapula and innominate bone [76]. Vultures frequently feed on body openings as anus, enlarge them, and try to reach internal organs through them. After consuming soft tissues of the head, they feed on cervical region and try to access into fatty brain tissue through foramen magnum. As a result, while vultures try to access into brain during feeding activity, cervical vertebras are consumed, and bone tissue around foramen magnum is damaged. Since intra-abdominal organs are tried to be accessed through anus, lumbar vertebras are frequently spared [5]. Asamura et al. presented two carbonized corpses. In their cases, crows had caused bulgings on head and extremities while they were pulling and stretching attached nerve fibers, tendons, and ligaments with their beaks during their feeding activities, and in one case, defective areas with serrated contours corresponding to the configuration of the beaks of crows in lungs, liver, spleen, and kidneys were found [62]. Behavior pattern of birds and bird species exerting scavenging activity demonstrate seasonal and regional variation [77]. In West Australia, the dominant scavenger bird is raven [4, 77], while in Arizona–Texas, it is the vulture [5, 39]. It has been determined that ravens prefer to feed on corpses at sunrise and sunset during summer months, while during cold winter months, they prefer to feed during hot daytime hours [77]. After scavenging activity of birds, bones and personal belongings of the deceased may scatter around a large area. It has been determined that vultures visit skeletonized corpse and scatter the bones after they skeletonize the corpse. It has been indicated that the vultures scatter bones and personal belongings 25 m far away from the first location of the corpse, so it has been suggested that in these cases area of investigation should encompass at least an area of 100 m^2 [5].

The common characteristics of postmortem wounds caused by carnivorous animals are the presence of lesions resembling stab wounds because of their canine teeth and frequently linear scratches created by paws near these wounds [2, 26]. Punctured, irregular, partially curled "V" or rhomboid-shaped wound edges in soft tissue caused by bites of Canidae (wolf, pet dogs, jackal, fox, etc.) are seen [7, 9, 10, 12, 25] (**Figures 7** and **8**). Canidae uses its mandibular and maxillary canine teeth during feeding and create punctures and multiple numbers of adjacent tears in the soft tissue caused by shear–bites, which are termed as "one hole-one tear" combination [81]. The animal uses this region as a fulcrum, counteracts the weight of the corpse, and rapidly shakes its head repetitively from right to left and vice versa to pluck the tissue and creates stretch-rupture defects [25]. Canidae may cause pit, puncture, score, and furrow-type bite marks on the bone surface [33]. Various breeds of dogs in the same family may have diverse teeth size, jaw, bite strength, scavenging behavior, and pattern, which affect the configuration of bite marks on the bone surface [82–84]. Carnivorous animals frequently cause destructive changes on epiphyseal ends of long bones; transverse and spinous processes of vertebras; and distal ends of ribs, scapula, and hip bones [33, 37]. Postmortem scavenging lesions caused by animals belonging to the Canidae family are most frequently seen in nose, mouth, neck, and upper and lower extremities and least frequently in anus, penis, and abdomen [25]. Wounds caused by animals belonging to the Felidae family have sharper and smooth edges just as cut by a knife, and on the edges of the wounds, linear, scratch-type lesions formed by paws may be detected [10, 29, 44, 85]. Rippley et al. [44] investigated scavenging behavior of bobcats (*Lynx Rufus*). They observed these animals for 32 days and reported that bobcats consumed

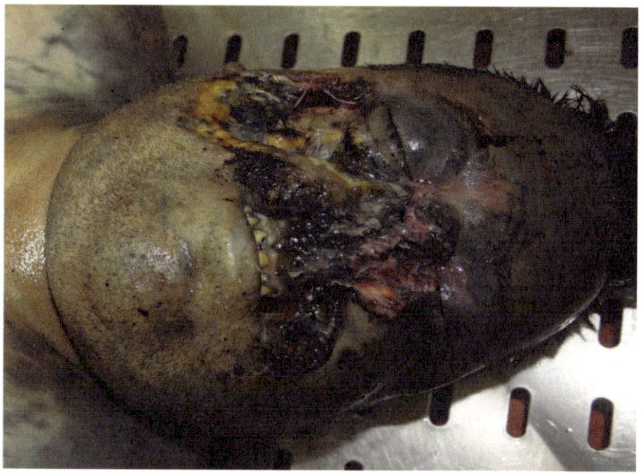

Figure 7. Common soft and muscle tissue loss on right cheek, nose, and upper lip due to postmortem Canidae scavenging (Archive of Council of Forensic Medicine, Turkey).

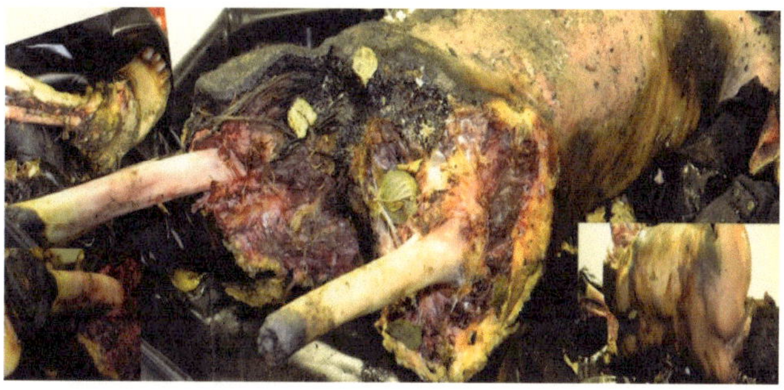

Figure 8. A corpse of a 17-year-old man who died because of stabbing and was burned after death. Amputated left limb, extensive soft tissue, and muscle loss that exposed bone tissue of lower limbs and hip caused by postmortem Canidae scavenging activity.

soft tissues of the forearms, hips, thighs, and abdominal region and left multiple puncture marks on the ulna and radius with an attempt to disarticulate the arm. Besides, it was demonstrated that lynx tried to hide the corpse with a heap of mud, grass, and pine needles after it consumed the corpse for future feeding process, which might create complications as for the identification of the corpse by forensic medicine and forensic anthropology. Bears are one of the biggest carnivorans, which cause postmortem injuries [40]. Carson et al. [40] indicated the presence of significant differences in scavenging models of bears and canid family and argued that discrimination between bears and dogs based on the presence or absence of remains of human skeletons found in and around the incident site is possible. Bears usually devour axial skeleton and tend to consume, extract, or damage vertebras, ribs, and sternum, while members of the canid family frequently damage extremities and through opened body holes devour internal organs incurring little injury on vertebral column. If only skeletal tissue was left behind because of scavenging activity of carnivores, the attacking animal may be identified looking on the length and width of the bite marks on the bone [33, 34]. It has been claimed that the average length (<2.5 mm) and width (<1.5 mm) of the pit created by red fox could discriminate the red fox from larger-sized members of the Canidae family [33]. Dominguez-Rodrigue and Piqueras [86] categorized the carnivorans based on pit lengths and widths they created on cancellous bone as follows: pit length < 4 mm, small-sized canines (jackals), and medium-sized Felidae (leopard and cheetah); pit length: 4–6 mm: (medium-large sized carnivorans (members of the Felidae family, excluding lion); pit length: > 6 mm: large-sized carnivorans (hyena and lion); pit width: < 2 mm small-sized members of the Felidae family; pit width: > 4 mm: hyena, bear, lion, and dog. Murmann et al. [84] suggested that when bite mark measurements of lower and upper jaws of animals are evaluated in combination, then discrimination between members of Canidae and Felidae is possible. Furthermore, Foust [34] claimed that when dimensions of bite marks and measurements of upper and lower jaws of the animals are evaluated in combination, then the species of scavenging carnivorans will be predicted accurately at a rate ranging between 75.5 and 78.3%.

Among scavenger carnivorans, pet dogs and cats that are responsible for attacks on corpses especially in indoor settings should also be mentioned. The wounds they create mislead the forensic investigator, and result in misinterpretation of the event as a criminal case. Postmortem attacks by pet dogs have been reported more frequently when compared with domestic cats [6, 7, 9, 10, 12, 17, 25, 27, 29]. When teeth marks of an animal were detected on a corpse in indoor settings, if on the incident site Pitbulls, Rottweiler, and German shepherd dogs are found, then the possibility of an antemortem attack should also be considered. Indeed, these dog breeds are "convicts" [49, 81, 87, 88]. It has been thought that pet dogs have regular food sources and do not feed on corpses; however, when they take a walk outside, they can also feed on corpses, and it has been indicated that in some circumstances, they may be unknown but important members of fauna consume corpses in the open air [5]. Antemortem dog attacks may cause wounds resembling those created by postmortem dog attacks. Therefore, signs of vitality on wound site, presence of bleeding, and results of histological examinations to be performed are very important in discrimination between antemortem and postmortem dog attack [21]. In indoor setting, attacks of dogs at corpse may start soon after death, in other words within hours [27, 28]. "V" shaped and rhomboid lesions occurred by the attacks of domestic dogs cause puncture-type wounds [9, 12], and domestic cat bites create small, round wounds with smooth edges [10]. Serious damages may be incurred on corpses leading to decapitation secondary to dog consumption of the corpse [12]. Bones and animal feces may be scattered all over the rooms of the home in scavenging activities occurred in confined places [6, 7, 9, 11, 12, 27]. The stomach of the offensive dog may contain personal belongings and body parts such as teeth of the victim that may be helpful in the identification of the corpse [12]. Chute et al. [7] presented a putrefied corpse of a 63-year-old female, and they detected amputation at the level of elbow joints of both upper extremities, diffuse soft tissue, and bone defects exposing underlying bone tissue caused by scavenging activity of a dog. X-ray of the Pitbull Terrier found at the incident site revealed radiolucent material (jewelry and teeth) in its stomach. From dog feces, 6 teeth, 3 earrings, and 10 finger nails were removed, which confirmed the identity of the corpse when compared with dental records. If the dog stays at home with the corpse for a sufficient time period, excluding a small part of the body or even a few bone fragments, all of the corpse may be consumed [6, 12]. In a case report presented by Steadman et al. [6], a 54-year-old woman who remained at home with her two dogs had died probably 4 weeks ago. When her corpse was discovered, only a calvarium and bone fragments of various lengths belonging to 60 different long bones had been detected. Rarely, it has been reported that in cases of death due to poisoning, domestic animals feeding on the corpse may be found dead at the incident site. Rossi et al. [29] presented a case of a 32-year-old male who was found dead at home, and tissue losses of his head, neck, and upper right extremity related to scavenging activity of a cat had been reported. Dead bodies of 10 cats of a victim had been also found at the incident site. Toxicologic analysis of the corpse revealed dothiepin intoxication as a cause of death, and the death of the cats had been also attributed to dothiepin poisoning.

In order to identify the species of the offending animal that demonstrated postmortem scavenging activity, it is very important to know scavenging animals peculiar to this region [5, 20]. Gunawarden [20] reported two cases taken out from water canal and two cases from the river in Sri Lanka. On various parts of the corpses, cuts, erythematous lesions, and soft tissue loss that did not demonstrate vital reactions without any bone defects had been found. Autopsies had disclosed the presence of postmortem wounds, which had been attributed to a large water monitor, i.e., kabaragoya (*Varanus salvator* salvator), and which is the second largest lizard after Komodo monster living in Sri Lanka. This animal has sharp claws; however, its claws and jaws are not strong enough to harm the bone. However, it creates cuts in soft tissues of the corpse as if formed with a sharp tools.

1.3. Postmortem animal attacks in water

If the corpse is immersed in deep waters, then it may be attacked by many sea creatures including fish, water rats, crabs, and amphipods [14–16]; however, if it is in shallow water, then predators living on land may damage the corpse [1]. In deep waters such as ocean and sea, many small fish species feed on corpses [14, 16, 89]. The best-known scavengers that feed on corpses in deep waters are sharks [1, 2, 89]. Shark bites cause clean cuts in skin and underlying soft tissue. Shark bites may cause flap-type elevations from soft tissue, which correspond to easily recognized triangular dental configuration of the shark [2, 17]. Besides owing to their strong jaw bones, they may cause extensive tissue defects together with fractures of underlying bone tissue [1]. If no one witnesses attacks of the shark, and only a part of the corpse could be obtained, then it is generally impossible to detect whether the wound is related to postmortem feeding or antemortem fatal attack of the shark [2, 17]. However, similar bite marks may be detected on clothes, and shark teeth buried in the bone can be found [90]. Byard presented a case report concerning the corpse of a 17-year-old male who had been drown, which demonstrated clean cuts and elevated triangular skin defects in the form of flaps on the left side of his neck, hips, and upper thighs caused by scavenging activity of a large-sized shark [17]. Teeth marks of the shark may change depending on the species and size of the shark. Hayashi et al. presented a case of a 50-year-old drowned female who had demonstrated circular, elliptic postmortem soyabean-sized (3.7 × 5.1 cm) wounds with relatively sharp edges on the anterior aspect of her neck [91]. They suggested that spoon-like concave bases of these wounds were associated with adipose tissue or superficial layer of the muscle, which were formed by cookiecutter shark (*Isistius brasiliensis*). These sharks are only 50 cm in length. With their thick lips and modified pharynx, they hold on their victims, and they rub sharp teeth of their lower jaw on the wound and create characteristic circular and concave lesions. Makino et al. presented a 60-year-old woman who had committed suicide and whose corpse had been found 6 days later in the ocean. The authors reported the presence of circular and "C"-shaped wounds on her corpse caused by a bite of a shark belonging to the Isistius species [92].

Relatively smaller fish can incur serious destructive changes in the corpse [1, 14, 16] (**Figure 9**). The most commonly known members of this group are piranhas [1]. Sazima et al. presented three cases of postmortem piranha feeding [93]. The first case belonged to a 25-year-old woman who had been found 4 days in a nearly skeletonized state after she had drowned. The second case was of a 50-year-old male. His corpse had been found within hours after he had been drowned with manifestation of diffuse loss of cranial soft tissue. The third corpse belonged to a 70-year-old male who was found 20 hours after he had fallen into water following a heart attack. The authors indicated that only a small amount of fresh flesh had been detected on his abdomen, while the remaining parts of his body had been completely skeletonized.

Crocodiles and alligators attack living beings with fatal outcomes and also assault corpses as well. Characteristic bite marks of crocodiles include holes pairing with each other and gradually getting closer to each other toward the nose [94] . Crocodiles have conic teeth and cause deep puncture and slash wounds [95]. Missing extremity parts and bone fractures including cranial fractures can be seen after attacks by crocodiles. Multiple punctate wounds with irregular edges can be seen secondary to crocodile bites [96].

Sea lice (*Natatolana woodjonesi*) are isopods nearly 2.5 cm in length that live on sand surface and in shallow waters. They move actively when they search for food [2]. Sea lice may surround corpses immersed in ocean very rapidly. Under appropriate conditions, they can quickly

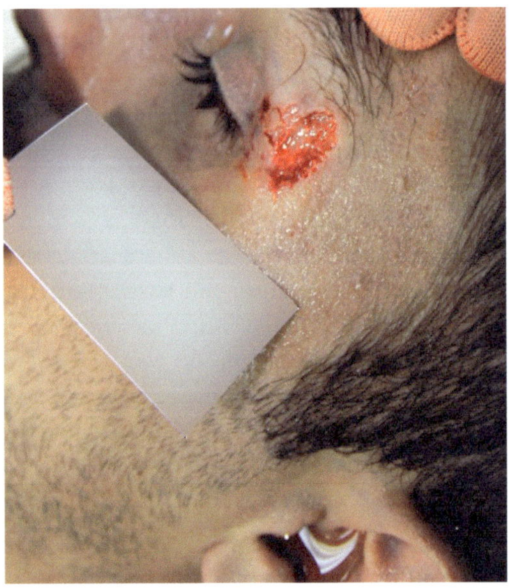

Figure 9. Soft tissue loss of 2 × 1 cm with semilunar-shaped notches of 0.1 cm in the edges due to postmortem small fishes scavenging on the left temple (Archive of Council of Forensic Medicine, Turkey).

multiply and open holes on the corpses, enter into subcutaneous layer, and devour muscle and subcutaneous tissue. However, the uppermost skin tissue remains intact excepting holes created [17]. Tsokos reported a case where sea lice caused a dramatic mutilation of the corpse's face within a short time as 12 hours [2]. Oval punctate lesions opened by sea lice so as to enter into subcutaneous layer may appear as shotgun wounds on exposed body parts such as the face [17].

Apart from fish, small sea creatures as amphipods, gastropods, and decapods also actively participate in postmortem scavenging activity in deep waters [14, 16, 89] (**Figure 10**). If in corpses taken out from deep waters, bones are not damaged markedly, and any bite mark is not detected on the surfaces of the bones, then the feeding of small sea creatures as amphipods, which easily move in tunnel-shaped clothes as pants, without displacing bones, and damage bone cortex, is conceived [16]. In deep waters, scavengers' consumption rate of the corpse may differ based on the depth of the sea where the corpse was found, latitude, and type of food [14]. It was reported that in North Atlantic a corpse of a whale weighing 50–100 kg found at 4000–8000 m deep might become a mere skeleton due to postmortem feeding within 15 days. Dumser et al. [16] presented case reports of two corpses belonging to one pilot who had a jet plane accident offshore of Namibia and another pilot whose helicopter crashed into the Mediterranean Sea. They indicated that in the Mediterranean Sea main scavenger species are decapods such as crabs and fish, while in the Atlantic Ocean, amphibians as lysianassid species are also involved in the scavenging activity, which speeds up consumption of the corpses. Just like sea lice, amphipods may invade all over the corpse and open tunnels in the corpse [14]. In addition, skeleton of the corpses found in deep waters may be damaged by gnawing of decapods such as crabs, apart from sharks, and great predators [16].

Sea stars live on the seafloor and cannot swim actively. During early postmortem period, sea stars cause development of hematomas by sucking action, which may be easily confused with antemortem hematomas. However, the discovery of a sea star on the corpse demonstrates that the corpse had remained at the seafloor for a while [2] .

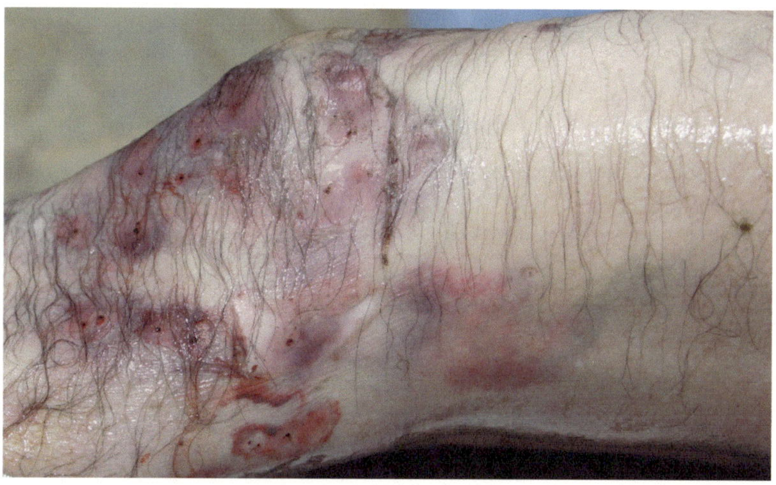

Figure 10. Oval, hemorrhagic lesions of 0.2 cm in diameter in the middle of red-colored ecchymosis of 1 cm in diameter due to postmortem small sea creature scavenging (Archive of Council of Forensic Medicine, Turkey).

Author details

Zerrin Erkol[1]* and Erdem Hösükler[2]

*Address all correspondence to: zerrinerkol@gmail.com

1 Department of Forensic Medicine, Faculty of Medicine, Abant Izzet Baysal University, Bolu, Turkey

2 Directorate of Bolu Forensic Medicine Branch, Council of Forensic Medicine, Bolu, Turkey

References

[1] Saukko P, Knight B. The pathophysiology of death. In: Knight's Forensic Pathology, 3rd ed., London: Arnold; 2004. pp. 73-76

[2] Tsokos M. Postmortem changes and artifacts occurring during the early postmortem interval. In: Forensic Pathology Reviews. Vol. 3. New Jersey: Humana Press Inc.; 2005. pp. 183-236

[3] Ozer E, Sam B, Tokdemir MB, Yildirim A, Cetin G. Medicolegal autopsy artefacts. Bulletin of Legal Medicine. 2010;**15**(2):68-74

[4] O'Brien RC, Forbes SL, Meyer J, Dadour I. Forensically significant scavenging guilds in the southwest of Western Australia. Forensic Science International. 2010;**198**:85-91

[5] Beck J, Ostericher I, Sollish G, De Le J, Desert S. Animal scavenging and scattering and the implications for documenting the deaths of undocumented border crossers in the Sonoran Desert. Journal of Forensic Sciences. 2015;**60**:11-20

[6] Steadman DW, Worne H. Canine scavenging of human remains in an indoor setting. Forensic Science International. 2007;**173**:78-82

[7] Chute DJ, Bready RJ. A case of postmortem canine depredation. The American Journal of Forensic Medicine and Pathology. 2017;**38**(2):100-102

[8] Byard RW. Autopsy problems associated with postmortem ant activity. Forensic Science, Medicine, and Pathology. 2005 Mar;**1**(1):37-40

[9] Tsokos M, Schulz F. Indoor postmortem animal interference by carnivores and rodents: Report of two cases and review of the literature. International Journal of Legal Medicine. 1999;**112**:115-119

[10] Tyagi A, Tyagi S, Malik N, Chawla H. Postmortem cadaveric depredation by animals – A diagnostic dilemma. International Journal of Forensic Medicine and Toxicological Sciences. 2016;**1**(1):20-23

[11] Weeratna J, Amararathna S, Rask R, Vidanapathirana M. Indoor postmortem animal scavenging. Sri Lanka Journal of Forensic Medicine, Science & Law 2014;**5**(1):2-8

[12] Buschmann C, Solarino B, Pu K, Czubaiko F, Heinze S, Tsokos M. Post-mortem decapitation by domestic dogs: Three case reports and review of the literature. Forensic Science, Medicine, and Pathology. 2011;**7**:344-349

[13] Tsokos M, Matschke J, Gehl A, Koops E, Puschel K. Skin and soft tissue artifacts due to postmortem damage caused by rodents. Forensic Science International. 1999;**104**:47-57

[14] Jones EG, Collins MA, Bagley PM, Addison S, Priede IG. The fate of cetacean carcasses in the deep sea: Observations on consumption rates and succession of scavenging species in the abyssal north-east Atlantic Ocean. Proceedings of the Royal Society of London. Series B. 1998;**265**:1119-1127

[15] Petrik MS, Hobischak NR, Anderson GS. Examination of factors surrounding human decomposition in freshwater: A review of body recoveries and coroner cases in British Columbia. Canadian Society of Forensic Science Journal. 2004;**37**(1):9-17

[16] Dumser TK, Türkay M. Postmortem changes of human bodies on the Bathyal Sea floor – two cases of aircraft accidents above the Open Sea. Journal of Forensic Sciences. 2008;**53**(5):1049-1052

[17] Byard RW. Diagnostic problems associated with cadaveric trauma from animal activity. The American Journal of Forensic Medicine and Pathology. 2002;**23**(3):238-244

[18] Tokdemir MB, Cetin G, Sam B, Ozer E, Yildirim A, Butun C. The challenges in autopsy cases exposed to animal attack. MediScience. 2014;**3**(2):1209-1223

[19] Haglund WD. Rodents and human remains. Journal of Forensic Sciences. 1992;**37**:1459-1465

[20] Gunawarden SA. Artefactual incised wounds due to postmortem predation by the Sri Lankan water monitor (kabaragoya). Forensic Science, Medicine, and Pathology. 2016;**12**(3):324-330

[21] Fonseca GM, Mora E, Lucena J, Cantin M. Forensic studies of dog attacks on humans: A focus on bite mark analysis. Journal of Forensic Medicine Science. 2015;**5**:39-51

[22] Willey P, Snyder L. Canid modification of human remains: Implications for the time-since-death estimations. Journal of Forensic Sciences. 1989;**34**:894-901

[23] Moraitis K, Spiliopoulou C. Forensic implications of carnivore scavenging on human remains recovered from outdoor locations in Greece. Journal of Forensic and Legal Medicine. 2010;**17**(6):298-303

[24] Campobasso CP, Marchetti D, Introna F. Postmortem artifacts made by ants and the effect of ant activity on Decompositional rates. The American Journal of Forensic Medicine and Pathology. 2009;**30**(1):1-4

[25] Colard T, Delannoy Y, Naji S, Gosset D, Hartnett K, Anne B. Specific patterns of canine scavenging in indoor settings. Journal of Forensic Sciences. 2015;**60**(2):495-500

[26] Shkrum MJ, Ramsay DA. Postmortem Changes "The Great Pretenders" in Forensic Pathology of Trauma: Common Problems for the Pathologist. New Jersey: Humana Press; 2007. pp. 23-64

[27] Rothschild MA, Schneider V. On the temporal onset of postmortem animal scavenging. "Motivation" of the animal. Forensic Science International. Sep 19, 1997;**89**(1-2):57-64

[28] Schumann M, Nolte I, Huckenbeck W, Barz J. Post-mortem animal injury – A few hours after death? Rechtsmedizin. 1996;**7**:22-24

[29] Rossi ML, Shahrom AW, Chapman RC, Vanezis P. Postmortem injuries by indoor pets. The American Journal of Forensic Medicine and Pathology. 1994;**15**(2):105-109

[30] Burkhardt S, Lardi C, La Harpe R. Postmortem partial skelitanization of the face and neck by an Appenzell mountain dog. Archiv fur Kriminologie. 2009;**223**(3-4):117-122

[31] Grellner W, Meyer E, Fechner G. Simulation of attempted homicide by dog bite in unconscious state. Archiv für Kriminologie. 1998;**201**:165-171

[32] Hayase T, Yamamoto K, Yamamoto Y. An unusual case of extensive cadaver ingestion by a domestic dog. Archiv für Kriminologie. 1994;**194**:177-181

[33] Young A, Stillman R, Smith MJ, Korstjens AH. Scavenger species-typical alteration to bone: Using bite mark dimensions to identify scavengers. Journal of Forensic Sciences. 2015;**60**(6):1426-1435

[34] Foust Jennifer L. The use of tooth pit and tooth/jaw measurements to identify carnivore taxa responsible for damage on scavenged bone. Graduate Student Theses, Dissertations, & Professional Papers 1102. 2010. Available from: https://scholarworks.umt.edu/etd/1102 (Accessed: Nov 20, 2017)

[35] Pickering TR, Dominguez-Rodrigo M, Egeland CP, Brain CK. Beyond leopards: Tooth marks and the contribution of multiple carnivore taxa to the accumulation of the Swartkrans member 3 fossil assemblage. Journal of Human Evolution. 2004;**46**:595-604

[36] Coard R. Ascertaining an agent: Using tooth pit data to determine the carnivores responsible for predation in cases of suspected big cat kills in an upland area of Britain. Journal of Archaeological Science. 2007;**34**:1677-1684

[37] Haglund WD, Reay DT, Swindler DR. Tooth mark artifacts and survival of bones in animal scavenged human skeletons. Journal of Forensic Sciences. 1988;**33**(4):985-997

[38] Selvaggio MM. Carnivore tooth marks and stone tool butchery marks on scavenged bones: Archaeological implications. Journal of Human Evolution. 1994;**27**(1-3):215-228

[39] Spradley MK, Spradley MK, Hamilton MD, Giordano A. Spatial patterning of vulture scavenged human remains. Forensic Science International. 2014;**219**(1-3):57-63

[40] Carson EA, Stefan VH, Powell JF. Skeletal manifestations of bear scavenging skeletal manifestations of bear scavenging. Journal of Forensic Sciences. 2000;**45**(3):515-526

[41] Haglund WD, Reay DT, Swindler DR. Canid scavenging/disarticulation sequence of human remains in the Pacific northwest. Journal of Forensic Sciences. 1989;**34**(3):587-606

[42] Kjorlien YP, Beattie OB, Peterson AE. Scavenging activity can produce predictable patterns in surface skeletal remains scattering: Observations and comments from two experiments. Forensic Science International. 2009 Jul 1;**188**(1-3):103-106

[43] Jeong Y, Jantz LM, Smith J. Investigation into seasonal scavenging patterns of raccoons on human. Journal of Forensic Sciences. Mar 2016;**61**(2):467-471

[44] Rippley A, Larison NC, Moss KE, Kelly JD, Bytheway JA. Scavenging behavior of Lynx rufus on human remains during the winter months of Southeast Texas. Journal of Forensic Sciences. 2012;**57**(3):699-705

[45] Lauridson JR, Meyers L. Evaluation of fatal dog bites: The view of the medical examiner and animal behaviorist. Journal of Forensic Sciences. 1993;**38**:726-731

[46] Clark MA, Sandusky GE, Hawley DA, Pless JE, Fardal PM, Tate LR. Fatal and near-fatal animal bite injuries. Journal of Forensic Sciences. 1991;**36**:1256-1261

[47] Salem NH, Belhadj M, Aissaoui A, Mesrati MA, Chadly A. Multidisciplinary approach to fatal dog attacks: A forensic case study. Journal of Forensic and Legal Medicine. 2013;**20**(6):763-766

[48] Patel F. Artefact in forensic medicine: Postmortem rodent activity. Journal of Forensic Sciences. 1994;**39**:257-260

[49] Tsokos M, Byard RW, Püschel K. Extensive and mutilating craniofacial trauma involving defleshing and decapitation. The American Journal of Forensic Medicine and Pathology. 2007;**28**:131-136

[50] Pollak S, Nadjem H, Faller-Marquardt M. Agonal dog bite injuries. Beiträge zur Gerichtlichen Medizin. 1992;**50**:351-356

[51] Ohshima T. Forensic wound examination. Forensic Science International. 2000;**113**:153-164

[52] Grellner W, Madea B. Demands on scientific studies: Vitality of wounds and wound age estimation. Forensic Science International. Jan 17, 2007;**165**(2-3):150-154

[53] Hernández-Cueto C, Girela E, Sweet DJ. Advances in the diagnosis of wound vitality: A review. The American Journal of Forensic Medicine and Pathology. 2000;**21**(1):21-31

[54] Dressler J, Bachmann L, Strejc P, Koch R, Müller E. Expression of adhesion molekules in skin wounds: Diagnostic value in legal medicine. Forensic Science International. 2000 Sep 11;**113**(1-3):173-176

[55] Dressler J, Bachmann L, Koch R, Müller E. Estimation of wound age and VCAM-1 in human skin. International Journal of Legal Medicine. 1999;**112**(3):159-162

[56] Balazic J, Grajn A, Kralj E, Serko A, Stefanic B. Expression of fibronectin suicidal in gun shot wounds. Forensic Science International. Jan 17, 2005;**147**(Suppl):S5-S7

[57] Pakis I, Kaya EA. Evaluation of vitality and wound age in forensic medicine practice. Journal of Forensic Medicine. 2011;**25**(2):137-152

[58] Grellner W, Vieler S, Madea B. Transforming growth factors (TGFalpha and TGF-beta1) in the determination of vitality and wound age: Immunohistochemical study on human skin wounds. Forensic Science International. 2005;**153**:174-180

[59] Hernández-Cueto C, Vieira DN, Girela E, Marques E, Villanueva E, Sá FO. Diagnostic ability of D-dimer in the establishment of the vitality of wounds. Forensic Science International. 1995;**76**(2):141-149

[60] Ortiz-Rey JA, Suárez-Peñaranda JM, Muñoz-Barús JI, Alvarez C, San Miguel P, Rodríguez-Calvo MS, Concheiro-Carro L. Expression of fibronectin and tenascin as a demonstration of vital reaction in rat skin and muscle. International Journal of Legal Medicine. 2003;**7**(6):356-360

[61] He L, Zhu J. Distinguishing antemortem from postmortem injuries by LTB4 quantification. Forensic Science International. 1996;**81**(1):11-16

[62] Asamura H, Takayanagi K, Ota M, Kobayashi K, Fukushima H. Unusual characteristic patterns of postmortem injuries. Journal of Forensic Sciences. 2004 May;**49**(3):592-594

[63] Pollak S, Reiter C. Maggot-induced postmortem changes simulating gunshot wounds. Archiv für Kriminologie. 1988;**181**(5-6):146-154

[64] Komar D, Beattie O. Postmortem insect activity may mimic Perimortem sexual assault clothing patterns. Journal of Forensic Sciences. 1998;**43**(4):792-796

[65] Prahlow J. Postmortem changes and time of death. In: Forensic Pathology for Police, Death Investigators, Attorneys, and Forensic Scientists. Springer Science & Business Media. 2010. pp. 162-184

[66] Anderson GS. Determining time of death using blow fly eggs in the early postmortem interval. International Journal of Legal Medicine. 2004 Aug;**118**(4):240-241

[67] Sharma R, Garg RK, Gaur JR. Various methods for the estimation of the post mortem interval from Calliphoridae: A review. Egyptian Journal of Forensic Sciences. 2015;**5**(1):1-12

[68] Davies K, Harvey ML. Internal morphological analysis for age estimation of blow fly pupae (*Diptera*: *Calliphoridae*) in postmortem interval analysis. Journal of Forensic Sciences. 2013;**58**(1):79-84

[69] Broen K, Thorne A, Harvey M. Preservation of *Calliphora vicina* (*Diptera*: *Calliphoridae*) pupae for use in postmortem interval estimation. Forensic Science International. 2012;**223**: 176-183

[70] Amendt J, Campobasso CP, Gaudry E, Reiter C, LeBlance HN, Hall MJR. Best practice in forensic entomology-standarts and guidelines. International Journal of Legal Medicine. 2007;**121**:90-104

[71] Chávez-Briones ML, Hernández-Cortés R, Díaz-Torres P, Niderhauser-García A, Ancer-Rodríguez J, Jaramillo-Rangel G, Ortega-Martínez M. Identification of human remains by DNA analysis of the gastrointestinal contents of fly larvae. Journal of Forensic Sciences. 2013;**58**(1):248-250

[72] Wells J, Introna F, Di Vella G, Campobasso C, Hayes J, Sperling F. Human and insect mitochondrial DNA analysis from maggots. Journal of Forensic Sciences. 2001;**46**(3):685-687

[73] Goff ML, Win BH. Estimation of postmortem interval based on colony development time for Anoplolepsis longipes (*Hymenoptera*: *Formicidae*). Journal of Forensic Sciences. 1997;**42**:1176-1179

[74] Ropohl D, Scheithauer R, Pollak S. Postmortem injuries inflicted by domestic golden hamster: Morphological aspects and evidence by DNA typing. Forensic Science International. 1995;**72**:81-90

[75] Erkol Z, Cantürk N. The problem of elderly people who live alone: An elderly neglect case. Turkish. Journal of Geriatrics. 2014;**17**(1):99-102

[76] Komar D, Beattie O. Identifying bird scavenging in fleshed and dry remains. Canadian Society of Forensic Science Journal. 1998;**31**(3):177-188

[77] O'Brien RC, Forbes SL, Meyer J, Dadour IR. A preliminary investigation into the scavenging activity on pig carcasses in Western Australia. Forensic Science, Medicine, and Pathology. 2007;**3**:194-199

[78] Dettling A, Strohbeck-Kuhner P, Schmitt G, Haffner HT. Animal bites caused by a song bird. Archiv für Kriminologie. 2001;**208**:48-53

[79] Hayase T, Yamamoto K, Yamamoto Y, Nishitani Y, Abiru H, Fukui Y. Analysis of postmortem injuries inflicted by animals and the environment. Acta Crim Japon. 1999;**65**:226-234

[80] Reeves NM. Taphonomic effects of vulture scavenging. Journal of Forensic Sciences. 2009;**54**(3):523-528

[81] De Munnynck K, Van de Voorde W. Forensic approach of fatal dog attacks: A case report and literature review. International Journal of Legal Medicine. 2002;**116**:295-300

[82] Gidna A, Yravedra J, Dominguez-Rodrigo M. A cautionary note on the use of captive carnivores to model wild predator behavior: A comparison of bone modification patterns on long bones by captive and wild lions. Journal of Archaeological Science. 2013;**40**:1903-1910

[83] Young A, Marquez-Grant N, Stillman R, Smith MJ, Korstjens AH. An investigation of red fox (Vulpes vulpes) and Eurasian badger (Meles meles) scavenging, scattering and removal of deer remains: Forensic implications and applications. Journal of Forensic Sciences. 2015;**60**:39-55

[84] Murmann DC, Brumit PC, Schrader BA, Senn DR. A comparison of animal jaws and bite mark patterns. Journal of Forensic Sciences. 2006;**51**(4):846-860

[85] Cohle SD, Harlan CW, Harlan G. Fatal big cat attacks. The American Journal of Forensic Medicine and Pathology. 1990;**11**:208-212

[86] Dominguez-Rodrigo M, Piqueras A. The use of tooth pits to identify carnivore taxa in tooth-marked archaeofaunas and their relevance to reconstruct hominid carcass processing behaviours. Journal of Archaeological Science. 2003;**30**:1385-1391

[87] Sacks JJ, Sinclair L, Gilchrist J, Golab GC, Lockwood R. Breeds of dogs involved in fatal human attacks in the United States between 1979 and 1998. Journal of the American Veterinary Medical Association. 2000;**217**(6):836-840

[88] Pomara C, D'Errico S, Jarussi V, Turillazzi E, Fineschi V. Cave canem: Bite mark analysis in a fatal dog pack attack. The American Journal of Forensic Medicine and Pathology. 2011;**32**(1):50-54

[89] Dahlgren TG, Wiklund H, Kallström B, Lundalv T, Smith CR, Glover AG. A shallow-water whale-fall experiment in the north Atlantic. Cah Biol. Mar. 2006;**47**:385-389

[90] Byard RW, Gilbert JD, Brown K. Pathological features of fatal shark attacks. The American Journal of Forensic Medicine and Pathology. 2000;**21**:225-226

[91] Hayashi T, Higo E, Orito H, Ago K, Ogata M. Postmortem wounds caused by cookie-cutter sharks (Isistius species): An autopsy case of a drowning victim. Forensic Science, Medicine, and Pathology. 2015;**11**(1):119-121

[92] Makino Y, Tachihara K, Ageda S, Arao T, Fuke C, Miyazaki T. Peculiar circular and C-shaped injuries on a body from the sea. The American Journal of Forensic Medicine and Pathology. 2004;**25**:169-171

[93] Sazima I, de Andrade Guimarães S. Scavenging on human corpses as a source for stories about man-eating piranhas. Environmental Biology of Fishes. 1987;**20**(1):75-77

[94] Harding BE, Wolf BC. Alligator attacks in southwest Florida. Journal of Forensic Sciences. 2006;**51**(3):674-677

[95] Gruen RL. Crocodile attacks in Australia: Challenges for injury prevention and trauma care. World Journal of Surgery. 2009;**33**(8):1554-1561

[96] Sinton TJ, Byard RW. Pathological features of fatal crocodile attacks in northern Australia, 2005-2014. Journal of Forensic Sciences. 2016;**61**(6):1553-1555

Chapter 5

Contribution of Forensic Analysis to Shark Profiling Following Fatal Attacks on Humans

Eric Clua and Dennis Reid

Additional information is available at the end of the chapter

http://dx.doi.org/10.5772/intechopen.71043

Abstract

Size assessment and species identification are paramount after a fatal attack for profiling a 'problem-animal' that could be specifically eliminated. In addition to ecological and behavioural data about candidate species, forensic analysis can provide critical information for achieving this goal. After providing basic information about fatal attacks and the anatomical features of the three species (white shark, tiger shark and bull shark) that are responsible for >80% of lethal interactions, this chapter presents the most used tools for assessing the species and size of a potential attacker. The size assessment can be done through measurements (on the body of the victim or from good-quality photographs) of the bite width (BW) and bite circumference (BC); the size is then obtained from regressions from the literature between BW/BC and total length. The average interdental distance (IDD) is also used through a similar process. Finally, other details of the wounds, such as the shape of the bite margin or of flesh flaps that directly depend on the jaw characteristics, can also be used to contribute to the final assessment. Although important, a forensic analysis should be complemented by data on shark ecology and behaviour for a more reliable conclusion.

Keywords: agonistic behaviour, shark bites, wound analysis, species identification, interdental distance, attacker total length, flesh flaps

1. Introduction: why profiling of sharks?

Although shark populations are facing declines worldwide, recorded instances of unprovoked attacks by sharks on humans have been increasing in recent years, stirring public concern and generating radical policies such as blind culling. The annual average number of fatal attacks increased from 4.3 persons per year (2001–2010) up to an average of 8.0 persons per year between 2011 and 2015 [1]. Such an unexpected trend can mainly be explained by a significant increase of the number of sea users that increases the probability of encounter between these marine predators and humans as shown in Australia [2]. In California, despite increasing records of white shark (*Carcharodon carcharias*) attacks, the individual attack risk for ocean users has decreased by >91% over a 63-year period (1950–2013) [3].

The triggers of shark attacks on humans are not well understood and still remain controversial. Such an understanding of attack motivation is jeopardized by the low number of attacks around the world, the scarcity of witnesses and the difficulty to observe an underwater event. A better understanding of shark motivations and behaviour through forensic analysis should at least partly help to avoid adverse outcomes in human encounters with these endangered creatures [4, 5]. If there is a witness to an attack, comparison of display features between the different species of potentially dangerous sharks can help in defining implications for shark-human interactions and suggests responses which may decrease the likelihood of attack for swimmers or divers faced with a postural display by a shark [6]. After the attack, the bite structure of the wounds may reflect the motivation and behaviour of the shark [7]. It can also allow the identification of the species involved in the attack and the accurate assessment of the animal size. The profiling (and potential elimination) of 'problem individuals' (see [8]) should be preferred to implementing inefficient blind culling of sharks (see [9]), whatever their species or size, as was recently the case in Western Australia and La Reunion island. In this French island of the Western Indian ocean, the decision to launch a culling campaign was adopted after five fatal attacks that occurred between 2011 and 2013; it not only removed tens of sharks (mainly tiger *Galeocerdo cuvier* and bull *Carcharhinus leucas* sharks) but also a white shark that was culled in October 2015, although this species is protected by international regulations. However, innovative solutions (to be set up in the near future) for spotting and eliminating the specific 'problem individuals' require early and efficient shark profiling after an attack.

The purpose of this chapter is to provide marine biologists or medical practitioners potentially involved in the postmortem analysis of a shark attack with the basic knowledge for assessing the species and size of a shark, based on bite features and tooth imprint. Our focus will remain on the data that should be collected and analysed from the wounds on a shark bite victim. This chapter does not include the ecological aspects (including life traits and behaviour of the sharks) which are a critical part of the holistic analysis of a shark attack in order to identify the shark species potentially involved in a fatal interaction. Neither does it include the problems that may appear when cadavers remain in the water for a significant period, creating several problems for diagnostics as shown by [10], nor forensic anthropology that examines taphonomic evidence of marine deposition and shark-feeding activities on human remains (see [11]). The focus remains on the postmortem analysis that can be conducted in the framework of an autopsy done in few hours that follow a fatal attack or the analysis conducted on photographs of the body, once quality images and suitable metrics are available.

2. Shark jaws as potential lethal weapons

Most sharks are predators that feed on other animals they capture, facilitated by adapted jaws holding several lines and rows of teeth. In contrast to mammalian teeth, shark teeth contain fluorapatite, $Ca_5(PO_4)F$, which is harder than hydroxyapatite [12]. Teeth may have different functions and thus different structures and hardness. For example, teeth of the mako shark *I. oxyrinchus* are curved to the interior and are used to puncture flesh of the prey, while teeth of tiger shark *G. cuvier* have serrated margins and are mainly used for cutting the prey in a sawing motion (**Figure 1**). The serrations vary from one species to another in coarseness and in distribution along tooth edges. Serrated teeth can make greater use of the available biting forces, and they have a greater cutting effect than do smooth-edged teeth (i.e. mako shark *I. oxyrinchus*). The latter depend upon friction which, because the coefficient friction is always less than 1.0 (often very much less), can make use of only a fraction of the total bite force [13]. However, smooth tooth blades can pierce prey with less resistance and are less prone to binding (becoming immobilized) in the prey tissue [12]. In carcharinids (including the bull shark *C. leucas*), heterodonty is characterized by triangular and serrated teeth on the upper jaw aiming at cutting, while teeth from the lower jaw are slender and smoother (see Section 3.4), acting as puncturing/holding devices before the shark starts moving the head laterally for cutting the tissues.

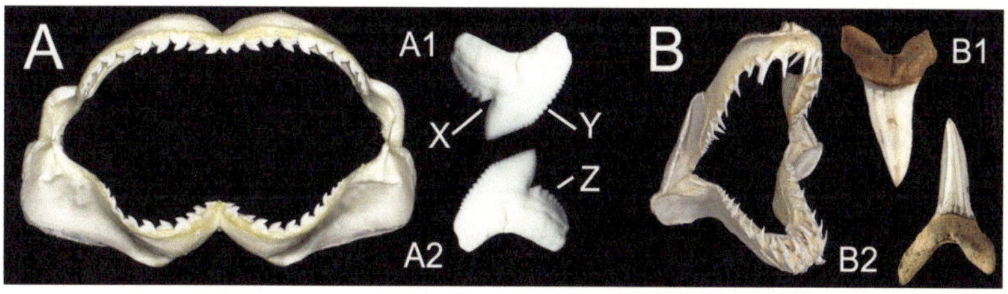

Figure 1. (A) Jaw of a tiger shark, *Galeocerdo cuvier*, showing the specific shape of the upper (A1) and lower (A2) teeth that are similar, showing homodonty between both jaws. The tiger shark tooth displays a strong distal notch (X), as well as fine serrations on mesial sides (Y) and coarse serration on the distal shoulder (Z). (B) Jaw of a mako shark, *Isurus oxyrinchus*, showing curved and thin teeth, smooth-edged without serrations, with a slight heterodonty between both jaws, teeth from the upper jaw (B1) being slightly thicker than those (B2) of the lower jaw (photos courtesy of Simon De Marchi).

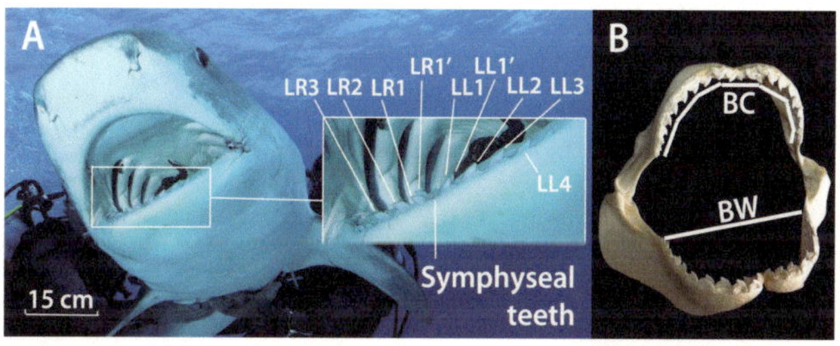

Figure 2. (A) Close-up of central lower jaw of a tiger shark, *Galeocerdo cuvier*, showing the specific shape and position of teeth from the lower jaw. Each tooth is named based on its specific position as follows: First L stands for Lower, second L for left and R for right. LL1, LL2, etc. constitute the first line on the left part of the lower jaw. Note behind LL1 and LR1, the replacement teeth (second row) (LL1′ and LR1′) that can be responsible for parallel teeth impressions. LL1, LL1′, etc. constitute the first row of the left part of the lower jaw. (B) Complete jaw of a tiger shark, *Galeocerdo cuvier* (photo courtesy of Simon De Marchi), that can be characterized by the jaw width, also called 'bite width' (BW), and the jaw circumference, more often named 'bite circumference' (BC). Both measurements can apply for upper and lower jaws, respectively (photos courtesy of Thomas Vignaud, left, and Simon De Marchi, right, for strict scientific use).

Whatever their sharpness and shape, these jaws and teeth constitute a potential threat to humans, also considering that certain species, such as the tiger shark, may produce biting forces of up to 3300 kg/cm^2 [14–16].

The dentitions of sharks are also well known for their ability to regenerate in a continuous conveyor-belt manner throughout life, displaying a high polyphyodontism [17], another characteristic of importance in the context of bite analysis. A tooth series is defined as the active teeth of a longitudinal jaw axis; a row is defined as the in-line teeth of any individual tooth of the active series [18] (**Figure 2**).

3. General features of fatal attacks on humans

3.1. Data for species most involved in fatal attacks

For the 370 shark species described, only 32 were documented as attacking humans, and 3 seem mainly involved in fatal attacks over the world: the great white shark, *C. carcharias*, accounts for around 50% of fatal attacks, the tiger shark *G. cuvier*, for around 20%, and the bull shark, *C. leucas*, for around 18% [1]. These three species are responsible for almost 90% of the fatal attacks, and this general trend is still prevalent. Based on recent outbreaks in Brazil (with 17 fatalities between 1992 and 2005) [19] and La Reunion island (with 9 fatalities between 2011 and 2016), the Bull shark *C. leucas* may pass the tiger shark as the second most dangerous species (**Table 1**). This chapter will focus on the features of these three species as the most probable candidates for documenting a fatal attack on humans.

3.2. The great white shark (*Carcharodon carcharias*)

The large, erect, strong, triangular, serrated teeth of *C. carcharias* allow a fast, high-impact piercing, slicing, cutting and fracturing needed when preying on large marine vertebrates [12] (**Figure 3A** and **B**). Head shape and musculature facilitate rapid lateral head movements in white sharks [20]. Over 70% of attacking white sharks are larger than 10 feet in length [1]. This is a reflection of the shift in dietary preferences of the white shark as it grows [21], moving from fishes to larger prey items such as pinnipeds, cetaceans and potentially humans when the shark approaches 10-feet total length (TL) [22].

White sharks exhibit a typical lamnoid dental pattern, with the upper dentition featuring marked heterodonty with slender teeth in the lower jaw [20, 23]. It is important to note that

Common name	Scientific name	Non-fatal unprovoked	Fatal unprovoked	Total
Great white shark	*Carcharodon carcharias*	234	80	314
Tiger shark	*Galeocerdo cuvier*	80	31	111
Bull shark	*Carcharhinus leucas*	73	27	100
Blue shark	*Prionace glauca*	9	4	13
Oceanic whitetip shark	*C. longimanus*	7	3	10

Table 1. Confirmed species of shark implicated in unprovoked attacks around the world (1580–present) (source: [1]).

http://dx.doi.org/10.5772/intechopen.71043

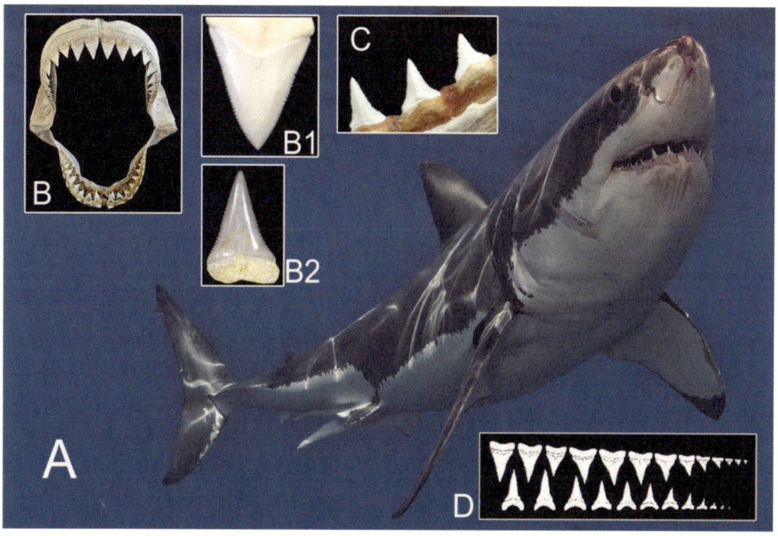

Figure 3. (A) General features of the white shark dentition, showing (B) a sigmoid pattern along a vertical axis of the jaw; anterior teeth are enlarged; anterior, intermediate and lateral teeth are compressed and form a continuous cutting edge; intermediate teeth are enlarged and over two-thirds the height of adjacent anteriors, with reversed cusps that are directed anteromedially. Jaws display a strong heterodonty with (B1) triangular upper teeth and (B2) slender lower teeth, as well as (C) large interdental gaps between teeth from both jaws (here the lower jaw) (photos courtesy of Douglas Seifert and Simon De Marchi for strict scientific use).

white sharks do not have symphyseal teeth [24]. The first and second anterior teeth (UR1 and UR2) of white sharks are erect and nearly symmetrical, while the lateral teeth (UR4 and UR5) become progressively slanted towards the jaw corner [25]. As described by [20], the upper dentition of white sharks features reversed intermediate teeth (UR3 and UL3) (see **Figure 4**). The reversed intermediate teeth (UR3 or UL3) create a significantly larger interspace measurement between it and the first lateral teeth (UR4 or UL4) than between any other two teeth of the upper jaw (**Figure 4**). Generally the large gaps that exist between teeth frequently lead to torn flaps of the skin and flesh between clear-cut punctures. These features should of course be taken into consideration when analysing a bite potentially from a white shark (see Section 4.3).

3.3. The tiger shark (*Galeocerdo cuvier*)

Both jaws have large teeth with curved cusps and finely serrated edges. Each tooth has a deep notch on the outer margin lined with numerous cusplets. Upper and lower teeth are similar in shape and size and decrease in size as they move back towards the corners of the mouth. There are 18–24 teeth in each jaw, these teeth forming a single cutting edge (**Figure 5**). The teeth have large cusps, forming a cockscomb shape, with prominent serrations [26]. The strong enamel cusps and serrations help strengthen the tooth structure and dissipate the biting stresses [27]. This makes the tiger shark jaw an extremely efficient and unique cutting tool [28].

The tiger shark is also unique because it has highly kinetic jaws that are exceptionally broad-based, heavily calcified and fused at the symphyses [29]. This allows for the single row of cusped, serrated teeth to extend out from the skull, seize the prey and begin to saw into the bone, performing the 'saw-biting' technique [30]. The broad, heavily calcified jaws, supported

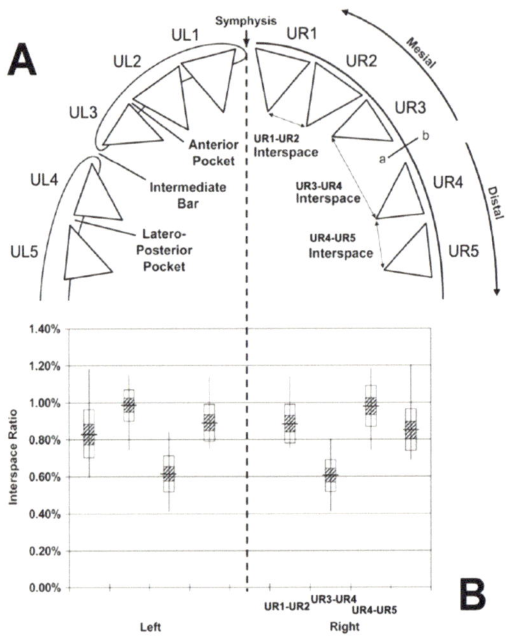

Figure 4. White shark dentition and terminology: (A) jaw terminology, tooth identification and measurements, showing location (indicated by chord a^b) of the intermediate bar between the intermediate (UR3 or UL3) and first lateral (UR4 or UL4) teeth, and (B) dice diagram of interspace ratio between successive pairs of upper teeth, where vertical bar1 = range, horizontal bar1 = mean, white box1 = standard deviation and hashed box1 = 95% confidence limits. In both (A) and (B), the vertical dashed line indicates head axis through the jaw symphysis (adapted from Ref. [20]).

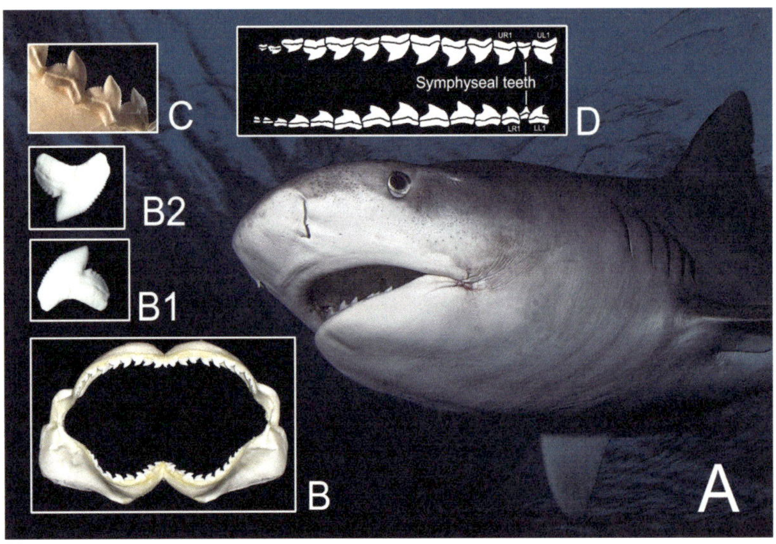

Figure 5. (A) General features of the tiger shark *Galeocerdo cuvier* dentition, showing (B) a sigmoid pattern along a horizontal axis of the jaw; teeth of (B1) the lower jaw and (B2) upper jaw are of similar shape showing homodonty (photos courtesy of Thomas Vignaud and Simon De Marchi for strict scientific use). (C and D) Right side of a typical tiger shark *Galeocerdo cuvier* jaw illustrating the single cutting edge formed by a single row of functional teeth (adapted from Ref. [31]).

by the extra-strong symphyseal fusion, reinforce the entire jaw apparatus and enable the shark to bite through very hard objects such as shells of chelonids [26].

3.4. The bull shark (*Carcharhinus leucas*)

Upper teeth of the bull shark are broad, triangular and strongly serrated, with erect or slightly oblique cusps, and their bases overlap with each other (**Figure 6**); lower teeth have a broad base and are narrow and slender with fine serrations, but no overlap with adjacent teeth bases. Usually, there are 13/12 rows of anteroposterior teeth in each jaw half, but they vary from 12 to 14/12 to 13 [32] (**Figure 6**).

As for many carcharhinids, upper teeth are primarily used to cut and saw (sideways movement along a surface when embedded in it, with ongoing perpendicular pressure); lower teeth are primarily used to puncture and hold prey item in position, with limited capability of cutting and sawing [7].

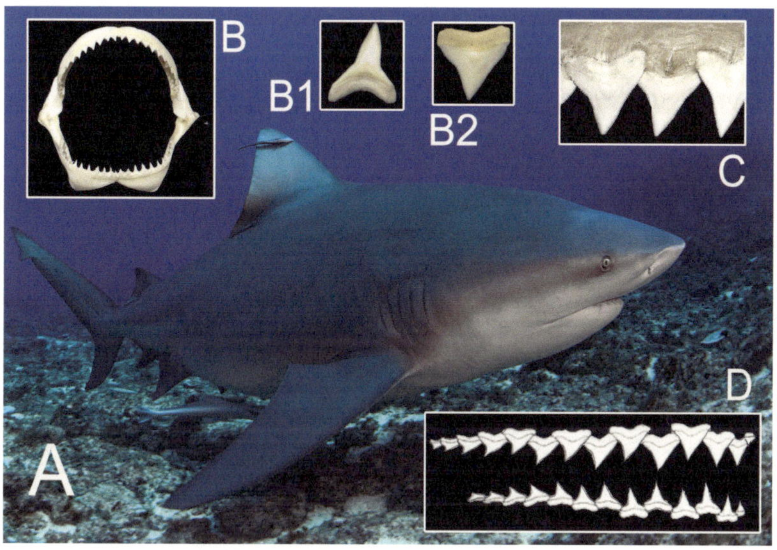

Figure 6. (A) General features of bull shark dentition, showing (B) upper and lower jaws; upper teeth (B2) form a continuous cutting edge with strong overlapping between teeth (C), while lower teeth (B1) are slender, displaying clear heterodonty. (D) Teeth from the upper jaw are usually more numerous than those from the lower jaw (adapted from Ref. [33]) (photos courtesy of Thomas Vignaud and Simon De Marchi for strict scientific use).

4. Post-mortem reconstruction of body length based on wound analysis

Along with the jaw and teeth features of the main candidate species, wound examinations usually focus on the number of bites, margin structure, tooth imprints, wound depth and tissue loss in order to assess the species identity [34, 35]. However, most of the time, these data are insufficient for a reliable identification and must be considered with ecological data about the presence and behaviour of the species (pelagic vs. coastal affinities, seasonality, etc.) and/or, if available, data provided by potential witnesses of the attack.

Historically, the size of the animal was assessed by comparing the length of the individual wound margins with jaws from known-sized animals [7]. Also, regressions that can provide the size of an animal based on the bite width (BW) are available (see **Table 2** for a review of regressions available from the litterature for white and tiger sharks).

However, inspired by studies conducted on cetaceans [39] and based on anatomical differences of jaws and teeth within shark species, Lowry et al. [40] proposed a forensic analysis method of shark bite wound patterns. It is based on the determination of a standard relationship between the measure of the average interdental distance (IDD) and the bite circumference (BC) of the jaw with the individual's total length (TL). The IDD and BC are allometric with the global size and are accurate predictors of the TL of a species-individual. Indeed, one of the numerous elasmobranch characteristics is a continuous replacement of the teeth throughout life, allowing the jaw growth. The number of teeth remains constant, but each new tooth is slightly larger than the one it replaces [41].

Thus, nowadays, in order to estimate length of a shark from an autopsy or file pictures, it might be rapid and reasonable to measure either interdental distances or bite radii from upper or lower jaws, whatever measurements are available, and apply them to established log–log regressions provided by [40] (see **Table 3**).

If the IDD and BC can provide critical information, they might be insufficient for a reliable result. It is therefore necessary to include other measurements of the wounds. Hereafter, we provide a series of case studies that indicate complementary tools that are available in regard to the situation and the available data.

Species	**Great white shark** ***Carcharodon carcharias***		**Tiger shark** ***Galeocerdo cuvier***	
Ref.	[36]	[37]	[38]	[39]
Regression	TL = (BW + 2.4642)/0.0986	BW = 10.4% TL +/− 1.3	BW = 11,7% TL +/− 1.7	BW = 0.12 TL +/− 7.99
n	6 (from 163 to 510 cm TL)	14 M + 19 F (from 170 to 391 cm TL)	10 M + 20 F (from 104 to 410 cm TL)	93

Table 2. Estimated total length (TL) from bite width (BW) for the great white shark and the tiger shark using regressions from the literature.

Type	**Jaw**	**Regression**	r^2	**p**
IDD	Upper	Y = 1.005x−2.111	0.98	<0.001
	Lower	Y = 0.925x−1.808	0.97	<0.001
BC	Upper	Y = 1.007x−0.800	0.98	<0.001
	Lower	Y = 0.966x−0.743	0.99	<0.001

Average interdental distance and bite circumference represent the dependent variables, whereas total length is the independent variable. r^2 = correlation coefficient; p = significance level.

Table 3. Log–log regression between average interdental distance (IDD) or bite circumference (BC) and total body length of white sharks, *Carcharodon carcharias*, based on [40].

4.1. The use of the bite width (BW) and bite circumference (BC)

Case study A: description of the wound on a 23-year-old female fatally bitten in a shallow water lagoon in New Caledonia. This case study was adapted from [42–44] *(same case).*

A single large bite was made to the right thigh, from the hip to the knee, with a length of 38 cm (**Figure 7A**). The thigh was cut deeply, with the femur bone broken at the level of the hip. The muscular mass was sectioned but was still attached to the femur bone whose distal part was still articulated to the knee. Despite the large bite, almost no tissue was removed as shown by the repositioning of the scalloped muscular mass on the leg (**Figure 7B**); the inner and outer margins on the wound on the inner part of the thigh fit together well although they are somewhat swollen. The blood vessels were divided, and according to the medical certificate, the victim died from exsanguination and hypovolemic shock. Apart from this large bite on the right thigh, no other wounds were identified on the body.

Given the size of the BC, the hypothesis of the bull shark was rejected to favour either a large white or tiger shark. **Table 4** provides regressions for these two species between the total length of the shark and the width of the mouth/jaw or that of the bite, from the literature. Considering the size of the bite width of 38 cm [44], the total length of the shark would range between 352 and 410 cm TL for a great white shark (for a similar bite width, a tiger shark would be between 250 and 383 cm TL) (**Table 4**).

Using a BC of 596 mm [44] and based on the regressions provided by [40], the species involved in this fatal attack seems to be a great white shark of about 3.5-m TL (**Figure 8**). However, these regressions also show that given a BW of 38 cm, the BC should be much lower than 59.6 cm for the attacker to be a tiger shark for which the TL would range from 250 to 383 cm TL (as shown in **Table 4**). The formula by [40] shows that a tiger shark with a 38-cm BC would have a TL >410 cm (**Figure 8**). This is due to the curvature of the BC which is different between the two species. The hypothesis of the white shark should then prevail. Also, based on behavioural features of the attack (provided by a witness), Clua and Séret [42, 43] concluded that the candidate species for this 2007 attack in Lifou Island was a white shark and not a tiger shark as supported by Tirard et al. [44]. This choice seems to be supported by the tools provided by Lowry et al. [40].

4.2. The use of the interdental distance (IDD)

As demonstrated by [40], the teeth sizes of some shark species vary directly with the total length (TL) of an individual, and a log-linear relationship exists between those two variables. The measure of the IDD can therefore give a reliable estimate of the TL of an individual for most species. The relationship between the BC and length gives a minimal estimate of a shark TL. It is less informative than the IDD because the marks left on the organism or object can be partials, as only a part of the jaw is often used during the bite.

The IDD is measured between adjacent teeth in the first six tooth files (a tooth in the functional row and its replacing teeth are a tooth file) on each side of the symphysis. It is the measure

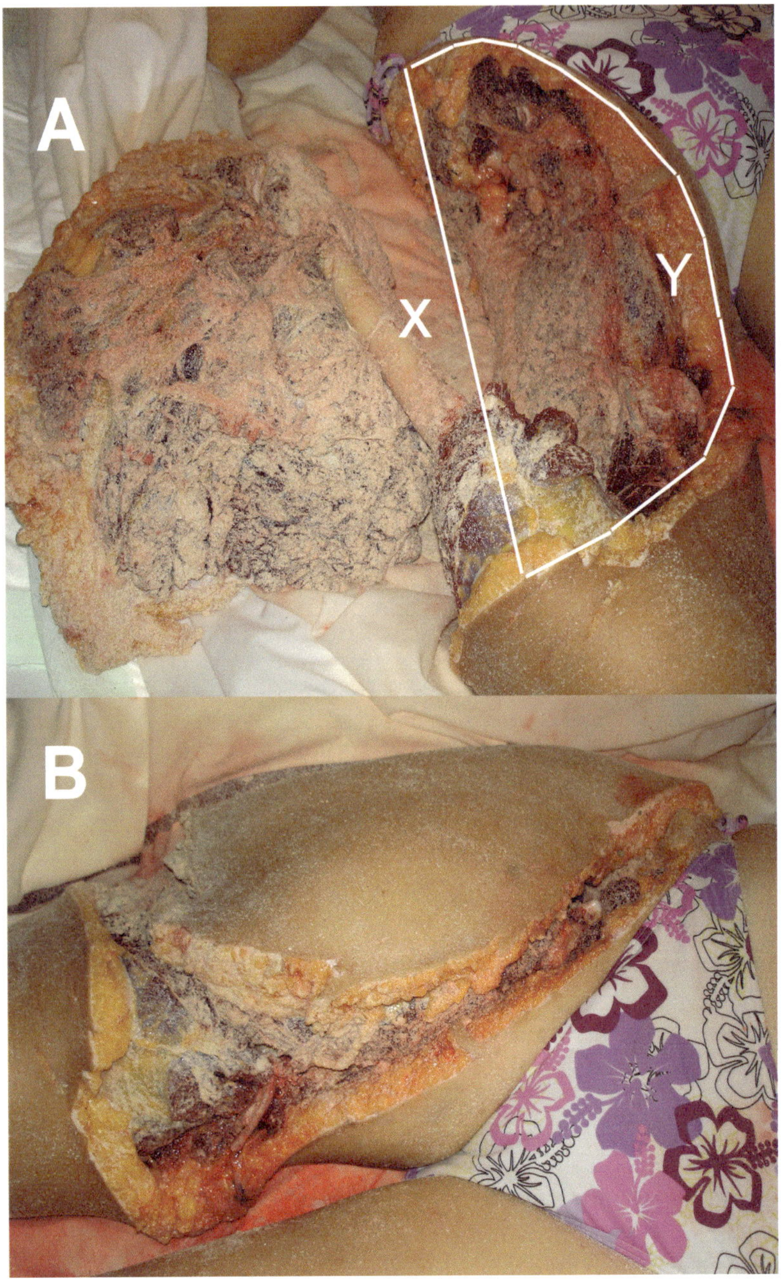

Figure 7. (A) Shark bite on the right thigh of the victim. X shows the bite width (BW) and Y the bite circumference (BC) that were accurately measured on the victim and used for the assessment of the shark size. The bite is not total; the thigh was not removed but is still attached to the knee; the femur is broken at level of hip. (B) The repositioning of the thigh scalloped by the bite shows that there was no significant loss of soft tissue (photos courtesy of Gendarmerie de Lifou for strict scientific use).

Species	Great white shark *Carcharodon carcharias*		Tiger shark *Galeocerdo cuvier*	
Ref.	[36]	[37]	[38]	[39]
Formula	TL = (BW + 2.4642)/0.0986	BW = 10.4% TL +/− 1.3	BW = 11.7% TL +/− 1.7	BW = 0.12 TL +/− 7.99
n	6 (from 163 to 510 cm TL)	14 M + 19 F (from 170 to 391 cm TL)	10 M + 20 F (from 104 to 410 cm TL)	93
BW (cm)	Calculated TL (cm)	Calculated TL (cm)	Calculated TL (cm)	Calculated TL (cm)
38	410.4	352.9–377.9	310.3–339.3	250.1–383.3

Table 4. Estimated total length (TL) from bite width (BW) for the great white shark and the tiger shark using regressions from literature.

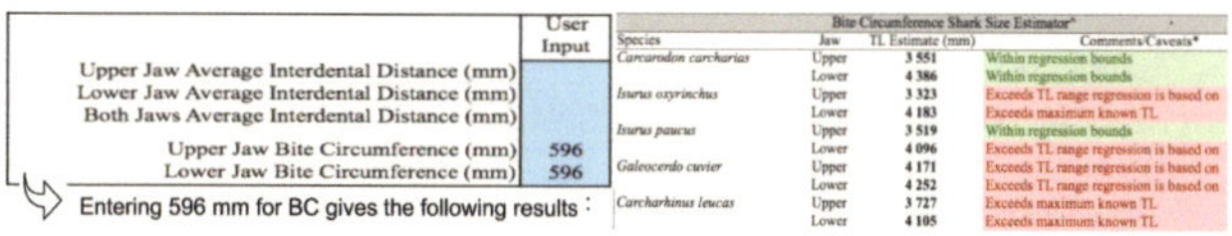

Figure 8. Screen copies of the results obtained through the excel table from Ref. [40]. In addition to the scientific paper, [40] provide as a supplementary material an excel table that directly uses the log–log regressions. You must enter either the average IDD or (in this case A) the BC for obtaining the potential species and shark size involved in the bite. NB: the comment 'exceeds TL range regression is based on' does not mean that the species cannot be responsible for the bite, but that the size is larger than the size interval of the sampled animals, indicating potential unreliability of the assessment.

between the tip of a functional tooth and the tip of the functional tooth of the adjacent file (see the interspace between teeth ends from **Figure 4**). The symphyseal teeth are excluded if present; they are often small, misshaped and randomly arranged. The IDD are measured on both sides of each jaw which leads to a total of 20 measurements for each individual [40].

Case study B: description of the wound on a 19-year-old male surfer who was fatally bitten on the outer slope of the barrier reef in New Caledonia (adapted from Ref. [45]*)*

Based on the body examination and the witness' declaration, it was evident that the shark attack was violent and sustained, with several strikes (> 3). Four main wounds could be distinguished: the right thigh was fleshless from the hip to the knee (with exposed femur), the right arm was missing, the right calf showed a large wound with no loss of tissue and a smaller wound was located on the right ankle which displayed clear cuts on medial and lateral sides that had dislocated the joint (**Figure 9**). The autopsy physician determined that death was probably caused by a cardiopulmonary collapse due to the huge haemorrhage on the severing of the axial and femoral blood vessels. To conduct the analysis of the wounds, we mainly used the 'interdental distance' (IDD) and the 'bite circumference' (BC) for assessing the species and size of the shark. Accurate calculation of IDD is actually easier with partial bites, and there was only one photo that could be effectively used for this calculation, showing at the same time a partial bite and a measuring scale (**Figure 9C**).

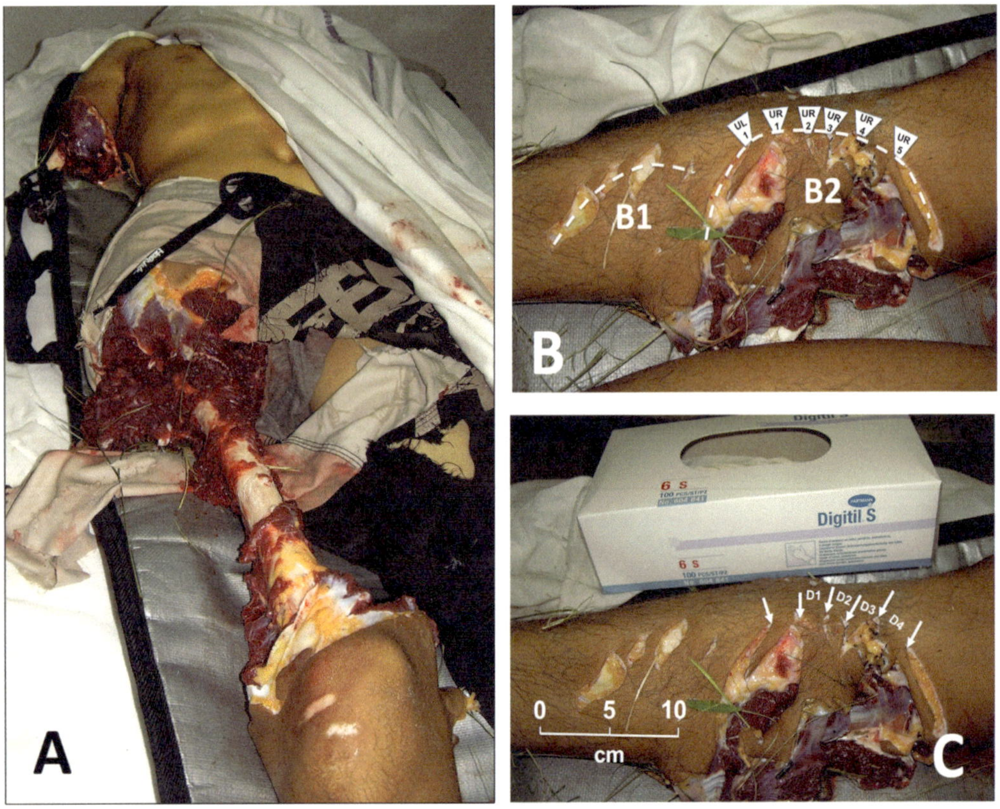

Figure 9. (A) The body of the 19-year-old victim showing the main two wounds in the right arm has been clearly severed 10 cm below the joint of the shoulder (top of the photo); all flesh and muscles have been removed from the right thigh, from the hip down to just above the knee (central and lower part of the photo). (B) Arcs B1 and B2 show the two main bites to the right calf, with tooth impression of the top jaw. For the left-hand arc (B1), it appears that the shark held the leg for a very short time, with a shallow holding bite, and then eased off before biting down and ripping with full force, just below the labelled marks (B2). On B2, we could define the first isolated tooth mark (top left) as the first upper left tooth (UL1), followed then on the right by the upper right teeth (UR1 to UR5). (C) The glove box (24 cm wide) gave us a scale allowing us to calculate bite width as approx. 17 cm, distances between UR1 and UR2 (D1) to be approx. 2.0 cm and UR2–UR3 as (D2) approx. 1.5 cm, UR3–UR4 (D3) approx. 2.4 cm and UR4–UR5 (D4) approx. 2.8 cm. The average IDD for the left bite arc is approximately 3 cm. The bite width probably represents the jaw width at the fifth tooth from the symphysis (photos courtesy of Gendarmerie de Bourail for strict scientific use).

The average IDD calculated on the partial bite of the right calf inflicted by teeth of the upper jaw of the shark (see **Figure 9B**) was 21.75 mm. Based on [40], only two shark species have upper jaw features fitting with such an IDD: a 2.65-total length (TL) white shark, *C. carcharias*, or a 2.25-TL longfin mako, *Isurus paucus*. The occurrence of a longfin mako off the reef barrier on the west coast of New Caledonia has an extremely low probability, as the species has a pelagic distribution. Furthermore, the features of the teeth marks on the body do not fit with elongated, thin and smooth-edged teeth (cf. *Isurus* sp.) but rather with large and serrated teeth with broadly triangular cusps, such as those of a white shark (*Carcharodon* sp.). We therefore concluded that a juvenile white shark of approximately 2.7-m TL was responsible for this fatal attack.

4.3. The use of other details

Besides the use of IDD and BC for assessing the species and size of the shark, the analysis of the pattern of the teeth marks, directly linked to the species-specific teeth characteristics of the shark, can also be compared with dental impressions of the three main candidate species. Rapid-curing vinyl polysiloxane impression material putty can be used to make these impressions using dried jaws from sharks of accurately measured total length (**Figure 10**). Such a process can help through the identification of specific marks and positioning of the teeth on the wounds, including the shape of tissue and flesh flaps that depend on the teeth position (see Case studies C and D).

Case study C: description of the wounds on a 15-year-old male kite surfer who was fatally bitten in a reef passage of the barrier reef of New Caledonia (adapted from Ref. [47]*)*

On the basis of the body examination and the witnesses' statements, it was evident that the shark approached the victim from below. A major wound (W1, 38 cm in length) with a significant loss of tissue was centred on both sides of the knee in the front and internal sides of the leg. Two other smaller wounds, with almost no loss of tissue, were inflicted on the back of the leg: one at the level of the thigh (W2, 18 cm in length and 10 cm in width) and another behind the knee and the top of the calf (W3, 30 cm in length and 7 cm in width) (**Figure 11**). As mentioned in the autopsy report, the death was undoubtedly caused by a cardiopulmonary collapse due to the huge haemorrhage following the severing of the left femoral blood vessel through the first wound.

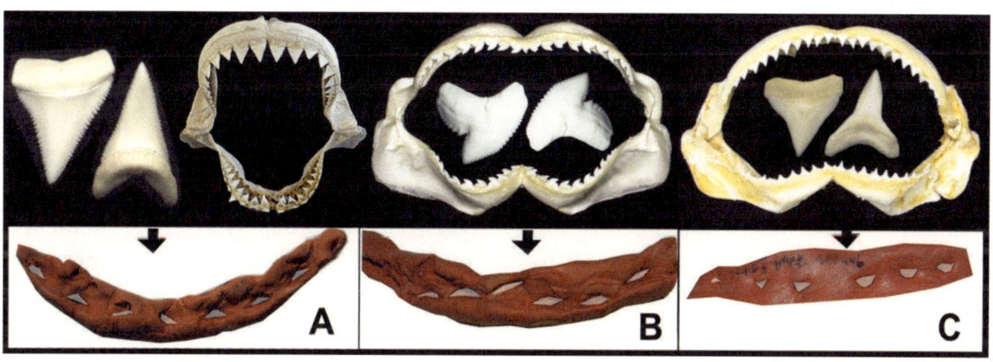

Figure 10. Teeth impressions from the lower jaw of the three main candidate species of shark, potentially involved in a fatal attack (from left to right): (A) white shark, *Carcharodon carcharias*; (B) tiger shark, *Galeocerdo cuvier*; and (C) bull shark, *Carcharhinus leucas*. The teeth impressions of tiger shark are long and thin, very close to each other, sometimes almost overlapping. Teeth impressions of bull shark and white shark are more 'needle-like' and separated, leading to much higher interdental distances (IDD) for a given size of shark. These jaws were collected from the NSW Shark Meshing Program [46] (photos courtesy of Simon De Marchi for strict scientific use).

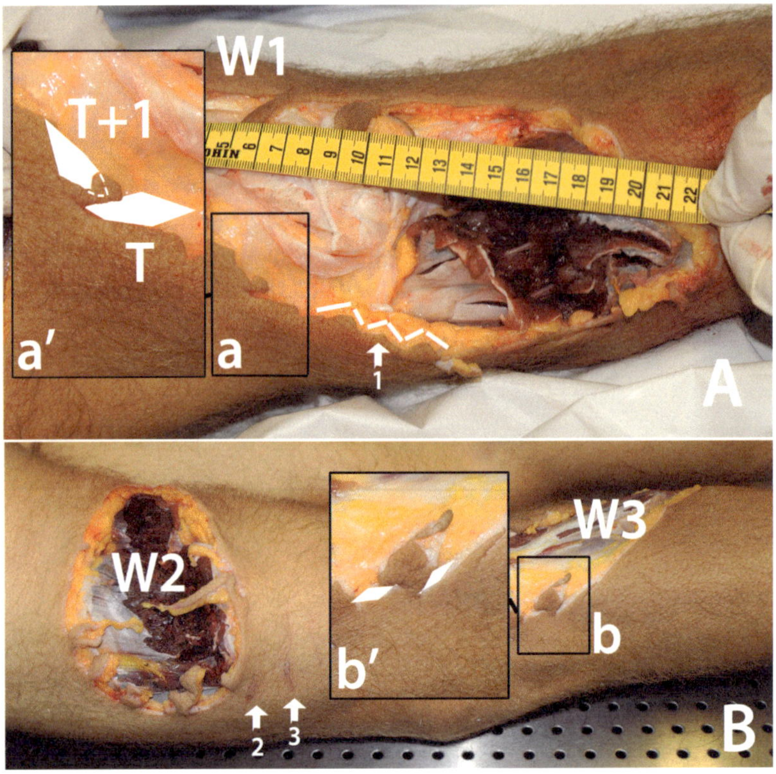

Figure 11. (A) Lateral view of the lower part of the first wound (W1). Arrow 1 shows the specific parts of the wound with sharp and square corners, quasi-parallel cuts, that are characteristic of a tiger shark teeth impression. (a') Close-up view on (a): showing a skin flap which results from two overlapping teeth (T and T + 1). (B) The third wound (W3) has an elongated frame with length 30 cm width 7 cm. (b') Close-up view on (b): showing a skin flap which also results from two overlapping teeth. Arrows 2 and 3 indicate two superficial scratches inflicted by two symphyseal teeth (at the junction of the two jaw segments) (photos courtesy of Gendarmerie de Koumac for strict scientific use).

The analysis of the first wound (W1) revealed that it was probably the result of two different adjacent and overlapping bites or one single bite inflicted as the leg was bending (see [47] for details). Analysis of the lower bite showed that the orientation of the tooth impressions and their shape, together with the small, smoothly sliced flaps, and the very smooth arc of the upper jaw bite, indicate a tiger shark as probably responsible for this attack. This hypothesis was confirmed by the observation of the three teeth impressions from the bottom left of the bite corresponding to this wound. These impressions are more or less parallel and have sharp cut corners, which is consistent with a tiger shark (**Figure 11A**). Also, the shape of the tooth impressions shows no clear morphological differences between those from the upper and lower jaws, indicating dignathic homodont jaws [47], characteristic of the tiger shark, compared to the white shark and bull shark which have dignathic heterodont jaws. In addition to these elements, the shape of some flesh flaps showed that there was an almost overlapping between the teeth (**Figure 11A** and **B**). This detail eliminates the white shark, and regarding the bull shark hypothesis,

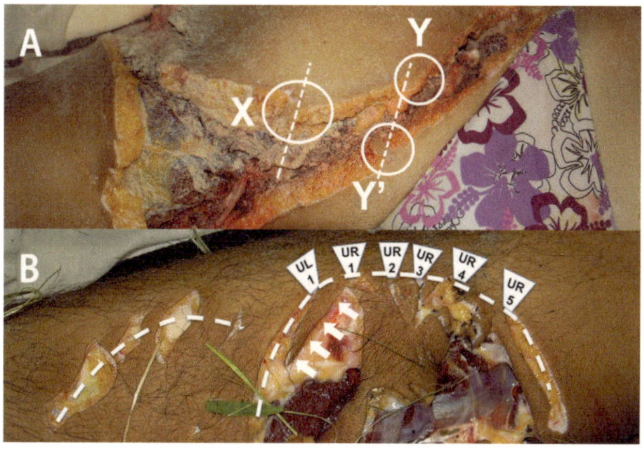

Figure 12. (A) Close-up of the wounds from case A that shows (X) a large flesh flap that seems to correspond to the symphyseal space of a white shark jaw, as well as (Y) and (Y′) flesh flaps that correspond to the large space that exist between UR3/UL3 and UR4/UL4 (see **Figure 4**). The dashed lines indicate the probable biting axis that can explain why both flesh flaps are not exactly opposite each other. (B) Close-up of a partial bite from case B, arrows show a large flesh flap that corresponds to the symphyseal space of a white shark jaw (photos courtesy of Gendarmeries de Lifou and Bourail for strict scientific use).

the overlapping in teeth of the upper jaw is so efficient (see **Figure 6**) that the presence of flesh flaps is unlikely.

Case study D: complementary wounds evidence for shark ID from [42, 45]

Case studies A and B also provide examples of evidence that support the identification of the attacking species. Actually, in both cases, the wounds presented large flesh flaps that are specific to the white shark, given the specific position of its teeth and the large interdental spaces (see **Figures 3** and **4**). In both case studies, it is possible to identify at least a large flesh flap that results from the space between the two first teeth of the upper jaw (UR1 and UL1), combined with the absence of symphyseal teeth (see **Figure 12**).

5. Conclusion

The present research aims at introducing marine biologists and medical practitioners to the basic knowledge necessary for analysing the wounds left by a shark bite. The implementation of these techniques is dependent on directly observing the victim or of the availability of quality photographs. Unfortunately photographic images often do not include any scale measure which significantly lowers the probability of an accurate conclusion.

In practice, these techniques can help but are often insufficient for species identification. It is then necessary to stress the benefit and utility of taking an interdisciplinary approach to forensic anthropological casework, specifically collaborating with a scientist with expertise in shark biology in cases of suspected shark attack. This type of integrated approach is common in taphonomic analyses and should be considered best practice [11].

Acknowledgements

In the context of case studies A and D, we wish to thank M. Neko Hnepeune, Mayor of Lifou Island; M. Dominique Mole, General Secretary of Lifou Island; M. Afif Lazrak, General Secretary of the administrative subdivision of the Loyalties Islands; and M. H. Ansquer, the vice-coroner of the French Republic in Noumea for trusting us in investigating the case. We also thank the parents of the victim for their understanding and her friend (L.L.) for her collaboration. In the context of case study B, we wish to thank the victim's mother, Rose-Marie Hannecart, for allowing us to conduct and publish this analysis. The file that allowed this analysis was kindly provided by the 'Procureur de la République', Tribunal de Noumea, Nouvelle-Calédonie, under the file reference 'Parquet/A0904702'; additional high-resolution images were provided by the 'Brigade de gendarmerie' de Bourail. In the context of case study C, we wish to mention that the file that allowed this analysis was kindly provided by the 'Procureur de la République', Tribunal de Noumea, Nouvelle-Calédonie. We also specifically thank Thomas Vignaud, Douglas Seifert and Simon De Marchi for the use of their outstanding photographs.

Author details

Eric Clua[1]* and Dennis Reid[2]

*Address all correspondence to: eric.clua@univ-perp.fr

1 PSL, Labex CORAIL, CRIOBE USR3278 EPHE-CNRS-UPVD, University of Perpignan, Perpignan, France

2 New South Wales Department of Primary Industries, Sydney Institute of Marine Science, Mosman, Australia

References

[1] ISAF. International Shark Attack Files. Website of Florida Museaum of Natural History. Available from: https://www.floridamuseum.ufl.edu/fish/isaf/home/ [Accessed 15-08-2017]

[2] West JG. Changing patterns of shark attacks in Australian Waters. Marine and Freshwater Research. 2011;**62**(6):744-754

[3] Ferretti F, Jorgensen S, Chapple TK, De Leo G, Micheli F. Reconciling predator conservation with public safety. Frontiers in Ecology and the Environment. 2015;**13**(8):412-417

[4] Caldicott DG, Mahajani R, Kuhn M. The anatomy of a shark attack: A case report and review of the literature. Injury. 2001;**32**(6):445-453

[5] Ritter E, Levine M. Use of forensic analysis to better understand shark attack behaviour. The Journal of Forensic Odonto-Stomatology. 2004;**22**(2):40-47

[6] Martin RA. A review of shark agonistic displays: Comparison of display features and implications for shark–human interactions. Marine and Freshwater Behaviour and Physiology. 2007;**40**(1):3-34

[7] Ritter EK, Levine M. Bite motivation of sharks reflected by the wound structure on humans. American Journal of Forensic Medicine and Pathology. 2005;**26**:136-140

[8] Linnell JD, Odden J, Smith ME, Aanes R, Swenson JE. Large carnivores that kill livestock: do "problem individuals" really exist? Wildlife Society Bulletin. 1999:698-670

[9] Wetherbee BM, Crow GL, Lowe CG. Distribution, reproduction and diet of the gray reef shark *Carcharhinus amblyrhynchos* in Hawaii. Marine Ecology Progress Series. 1997;**151**: 181-189

[10] Byard RW, James RA, Gilbert JD. Diagnostic problems associated with cadaveric trauma from animal activity. The American Journal of Forensic Medicine and Pathology. 2002;**23**(3): 238-244

[11] Stock MK, Winburn A, Burgess GH. Skeletal indicators of shark feeding on human remains: Evidence from Florida forensic anthropology cases. Journal of Forensic Sciences. 2017; DOI: 10.1111/1556-4029.13470

[12] Frazzetta TH. The mechanics of cutting and the form of shark teeth (Chondrichthyes, Elasmobranchii). Zoomorphology. 1988;**108**(2):93-107

[13] Enax J, Prymak O, Raabe D, Epple M. Structure, composition, and mechanical properties of shark teeth. Journal of Structural Biology. 2012;**178**(3):290-299

[14] Byard RW, Wick R, Simpson E, Gilbert JD. The pathological features and circumstances of death of lethal crush/traumatic asphyxia in adults—A 25-year study. Forensic Science International. 2006;**159**(2):200-205

[15] Whitenack LB, Motta PJ. Performance of shark teeth during puncture and draw: Implications for the mechanics of cutting. Biological Journal of the Linnean Society. 2010;**100**(2): 271-286

[16] Wroe S, Huber DR, Lowry M, McHenry C, Moreno K, Clausen P, Summers AP. Three-dimensional computer analysis of white shark jaw mechanics: How hard can a great white bite? Journal of Zoology. 2008;**276**(4):336-342. DOI: 10.1111/j.1469-7998.2008.00494.x

[17] Rasch LJ, Martin KJ, Cooper RL, Metscher BD, Underwood CJ, Fraser GJ. An ancient dental gene set governs development and continuous regeneration of teeth in sharks. Developmental Biology. 2016;**415**(2):347-370

[18] Nambiar P, Brown KA, Bridges TE. Forensic implications of the variation in morphology of marginal serrations on the teeth of the great white shark. The Journal of Forensic Odonto-Stomatology. 1996;**14**(1):2-8

[19] Hazin FH, Burgess GH, Carvalho FC. A shark attack outbreak off Recife, Pernambuco, Brazil: 1992–2006. Bulletin of Marine Science. 2008;**82**(2):199-212

[20] Martin RA, Hammerschlag N, Collier RS, Fallows C. Predatory behaviour of white sharks (*Carcharodon carcharias*) at Seal Island, South Africa. Journal of the Marine Biological Association of the United Kingdom. 2005;**85**(5):1121-1136

[21] Estrada JA, Rice AN, Natanson LJ, Skomal GB. Use of isotopic analysis of vertebrae in reconstructing ontogenetic feeding ecology in white sharks. Ecology. 2006;**87**(4):829-834

[22] Clua E, Guiart J. Sharks of Oceania: Ethno-ecology of a Marine Predator. 2nd ed. Papeete: Te Pito o te Fenua. 198 p; 978-2-9539509-8-4

[23] Shimada K. The relationship between tooth size and total body length in the white shark, *Carcharodon carcharias* (Lamniformes: Lamnidae). Journal of Fossil Research. 2002;**35**:28-33

[24] Hubbell G. Using tooth structure to determine the evolutionary history of the white shark. In: Klimley AP, Ainley DG, Editors. Great White Sharks: The Biology of Carcharodon carcharias. San Diego: Academic Press; 1996. p. 9-18

[25] Bass AJ, D'Aubrey JD, Kistnasamy N. Sharks of the east coast of southern Africa. 4. The families Odontaspididae, Isuridae, Cetorhinidae, Alopiidae, Orectolobidae and Rhiniodontodae. In: Investigational Report No. 39. Durban: Oceanographic Research Institute; 1975. p. 1-102

[26] Witzell WN. Selective predation on large cheloniid sea turtles by tiger sharks (*Galeocerdo cuvier*). Japanese Journal of Herpetology. 1987;**12**(1):22-29

[27] Preuschoft H, Reif WE, Muller WH. Funktionsanpassungen in Form and Struktur an Haifischzahnen. Zeitschrift fur Anatomie und Entwicklungs Geschichte. 1974;**143**:315-344

[28] Corn KA, Farina SC, Brash J, Summers AP. Modelling tooth–prey interactions in sharks: The importance of dynamic testing. Royal Society Open Science. 2016;**3**(8):160141

[29] Moss SA. The feeding mechanism of sharks of the family Carcharhinidae. Journal of Zoology. 1972;**167**(4):423-436

[30] Clua E, Read T, Chauvet C, Werry J, Lee SY. Behavioural patterns of a Tiger Shark (*Galeocerdo cuvier*) feeding aggregation on a whale carcass in Prony bay, New Caledonia. Marine and Freshwater Physiology and Behaviour. 2013;**46**(1):1-20. DOI: 10.1080/10236244.2013.773127

[31] Bigelow HB, Schroeder WC. Fishes of the western north Atlantic sharks. Memoirs, Sears Foundation for Marine Research. 1948;**1**:53-567

[32] Compagno LJ. FAO species catalogue. Vol. 4. Sharks Of The World. An annotated and illustrated catalogue of the shark species known to date. Part. 2: Carcharhiniformes. FAO Fish synop. **125**:250-655.

[33] Garrick JAF. Sharks of the genus *Carcharhinus*. NOAA Tech. Rep. NMFS Circ. 1982; **445**:194

[34] Davies DH, Campbell GD. The aetiology, clinical pathology and treatment of shark attack. Journal of the Royal Naval Medical Service. 1961;**48**:110-136

[35] Byard RW, Gilbert JD, Brown K. Pathologic features of fatal shark attacks. The American Journal of Forensic Medicine and Pathology. 2000;**21**(3):225-229

[36] Long DJ, Jones RE. White shark predation and scavenging on cetaceans in the eastern North Pacific Ocean. In: Klimley AP, Ainley DG, editors. Great White Sharks. The Biology of *Carcharodon carcharias*. Academic Press: San Diego. 1996. p. 293-307

[37] Bass AJ, D'Aubrey JD, Kistnasamy N. Sharks of the east coast of southern Africa. 3. The families Carcharhinidae and Sphyrnidae. Investigational Report No. 38. Durban: Oceanographic Research Institute; 1975. p. 1-100

[38] Heithaus M. Shark attacks on bottlenose dolphins (*Tursiop aduncus*) in Shark Bay, Western Australia: Attack rate, bite scar frequencies, and attack seasonality. Marine Mammal Science. 2001;**17**(3):526-539

[39] George JC, Philo LM, Hazard K, Withrow D, Carroll GM, Suydam R. Frequency of killer whale (*Orcinus orca*) attacks and ship collisions based on scarring on bowhead whales (*Balaena mysticetus*) of the Bering-Chukchi-Beaufort Seas stock. Arctic. 1994;**47**:247-255

[40] Lowry D, de Castro ALF, Mara K, Whitenack LB, Delius B, Burgess GH, Motta P. Determining shark size from forensic analysis of bite damage. Marine Biology 2009;**156**(12): 2483

[41] Moss SA. Shark feeding mechanisms. Oceanus. 1981/1982;**24**:23-29

[42] Clua E, Séret B. Unprovoked fatal shark attack in Lifou island (Loyalty Islands, New Caledonia, South Pacific) by a Great White Shark, *Carcharodon carcharias*. The American Journal of Forensic Medicine and Pathology. 2010;**31**(3):281-286

[43] Clua E, Séret B. Species identification of the shark involved in the 2007 Lifou fatal attack on a swimmer: A reply to Tirard et al. (2015). Journal of Forensic and Legal Medicine. 2016;**40**:58-60

[44] Tirard P, Maillaud C, Borsa P. Fatal tiger shark, *Galeocerdo cuvier* attack in New Caledonia erroneously ascribed to great white shark, *Carcharodon carcharias*. Journal of Forensic and Legal Medicine. 2015;**33**:68-70

[45] Clua E, Reid D. Features and motivation of a fatal attack by a juvenile white shark, *Carcharodon carcharias*, on a young male surfer in New Caledonia (South Pacific). Journal of Forensic and Legal Medecine. 2013;**20**(5):551-554. DOI: 10.1016/j.jflm.2013.03.009

[46] Reid D, Robbins R, Peddemors V. Decadal trends in shark catches and effort from the New South Wales, Australia, Shark Meshing Program 1950-2010. Marine and Freshwater Research. 2011;**62**:676-693

[47] Clua E, Bescond PM, Reid D. Fatal attack by a juvenile tiger shark, *Galeocerdo cuvier*, on a young male kitesurfer in a reef passage of New Caledonia (South Pacific). Journal of Forensic and Legal Medicine. 2014;**25**:67-70

Chapter 6

Defining Dental Age for Chronological Age Determination

Fatma Deniz Uzuner, Emine Kaygısız and
Nilüfer Darendeliler

Additional information is available at the end of the chapter

http://dx.doi.org/10.5772/intechopen.71699

Abstract

Dental age assessment is one of the most reliable methods of chronological age estimation used for criminal, forensic and anthropologic purposes. Visual, radiographic, chemical and histological techniques can be used for dental age estimation. Visual method is based on the sequence of eruption of the teeth and morphological changes that are caused due to function such as attrition, changes in color that are indicators of aging. Radiographs of the dentition can be used to determine the stage of dental development of the teeth from initial mineralization of a tooth, crown formation to root apex maturation. Histological methods require the preparation of the tissues for detailed microscopic examination. The chemical analysis of dental hard tissues determines alterations in ion levels with age, whereas the histological and chemical methods are invasive methods requiring extraction/sectioning of the tooth. In this chapter, the different techniques and considered studies were overviewed in conjunction with their advantages and disadvantages. It needs to be taken into consideration that rather than restricting on one age estimation technique, using the other available techniques additionally and performing repetitive measurements may be beneficial for accurate age estimation.

Keywords: chronologic age estimation, dental maturation, dental age

1. Introduction

Determination of the age is of great importance for the identification of unknown bodies or skeletal remains in forensics and anthropology [1]. In postmortem examination, the quality and quantity of the mortal remains such as the time passed between autopsy and death, environmental conditions and structure of the bodily remains or skeletal parts are critical factors. Additionally, it may also depend on other case-specific factors, such as costs, the time and equipment required.

For the age estimation, considering those critical factors, there are several methods available. Teeth can act as a biological marker of aging [2]. Teeth have highly mineralized structure, which makes them resistant to the postmortem decomposition and generally withstand flames, alkalis or acids [3]. Even bone may disintegrate, but teeth can be preserved for a long time and thus can be used reliably for identification in disaster situations [4].

Dental maturity is one of the most reliable indicators of chronological age estimation method used for criminal, forensic and anthropologic purposes [5–8]. Visual, radiographic, chemical and histological techniques can be used for dental age estimation [1, 9–11]. In this chapter, the stages of tooth formation/maturation, the chronology of tooth eruption and its relationship to age will be explained in detail. Methods of dental age estimation will be defined with their strength and limitations. The factors that may affect the dental maturation will be evaluated.

2. Chronology of tooth development

The development of the dentition is a continuous process that extends from embryonic to early adult life and it may be divided into a number of stages.

The sequence of prenatal mineralization in the deciduous teeth starts with the central incisor followed by the first molar, lateral incisor, canine and second molar. The maxillary central incisors and first molars are usually seen before those in the mandible. The lateral incisor appears first in the maxilla, but subsequent development is ahead in the mandible. Mineralization occurs in the mandibular canine before that in the maxilla, but it occurs simultaneously in the maxillary and mandibular second molars (**Table 1**) [12].

At the beginning of mineralization, tooth germs may be visible as radiolucent areas on the radiograph up to 6 months. A radiograph of the fetus taken at 26 weeks of intrauterine life shows advanced mineralization in mandibular anterior teeth. The mineralized outline for the

Tooth	Calcification begins		Crown completed		Eruption		Root completed	
	Maxillary	Mandibular	Maxillary	Mandibular	Maxillary	Mandibular	Maxillary	Mandibular
Central	14 wk in utero	14 wk in utero	11/2 mo	21/2 mo	10 mo	8 mo	11/2 yr	11/2 yr
Lateral	16 wk in utero	16 wk in utero	21/2 mo	3 mo	11 mo	13 mo	2 yr	11/2 yr
Canine	17 wk in utero	17 wk in utero	9 mo	9 mo	19 mo	20 mo	31/4 yr	31/4 yr
First molar	15 wk in utero	15 wk in utero	6 mo	51/2 mo	16 mo	16 mo	21/2 yr	21/4 yr
Second molar	19 wk in utero	18 wk in utero	11 mo	10 mo	29 mo	27 mo	3 yr	3 yr

Table 1. Chronology of deciduous tooth development mentioned by Proffit et al [12].

two cusps of the deciduous first molar, the one cusp outline for the deciduous second molar and the crypt of permanent first molar are seen [13, 14] . At 30 weeks of intrauterine life, mandibular anterior teeth shows 3/5 crown completion and the deciduous first molar cusps show fusion. The deciduous second molar with five cusps is seen, while no mineralization in the permanent first molar is observed. While the radiograph of the newly born fetus shows completely fused cusps for the deciduous first and second molar, for the deciduous second molar, there is no continuity across the occlusal surface [15]. At 32 weeks, the first permanent molars start to mineralize [12].

By birth, the deciduous incisors have about 60–80% of their crowns complete and canine crowns are a simple conical shape and approximately 30% fully formed [9]. The first deciduous molars have a complete occlusal cap of mineralized tissue, the maxillary tooth being more fully calcified than the other molars.

The eruption sequence of deciduous teeth in oral cavity is as follows: first, the mandibular central incisors erupt followed by other incisors. After 3–4 months, the mandibular and maxillary first molars erupt, followed, in another 3 or 4 months, by the maxillary and mandibular canines. The deciduous dentition is completed at 24–30 months as the second molars in both jaws erupt [12]. By the age of about 3 years, the deciduous dentition has emerged into the mouth and completed root formation (**Table 1**).

The transition from the deciduous to the permanent dentition is summarized in **Table 2** [12].

Except the third molars, all of the permanent teeth eruption takes place in two stages, between the ages of about 6 and 8 years followed by a silent period and again between 10 and 12 years. The first active stage begins at about age 6 with the eruption of the first permanent molars behind the second deciduous molar followed by the permanent incisors. The general eruption sequence is the mandibular central incisor, followed by the maxillary central and the mandibular

Tooth	Calcification begins		Crown completed		Eruption		Root completed	
	Maxillary	Mandibular	Maxillary	Mandibular	Maxillary	Mandibular	Maxillary	Mandibular
Central	3 mo	3 mo	41/2 yr	31/2 yr	71/4 yr	61/4 yr	101/2 yr	91/2 yr
Lateral	11 mo	3 mo	51/2 yr	4 yr	81/4 yr	71/2 yr	11 yr	10 yr
Canine	4 mo	4 mo	6 yr	53/4 yr	111/2 yr	101/2 yr	131/2 yr	123/4 yr
First premolar	20 mo	22 mo	7 yr	63/4 yr	101/4 yr	101/2 yr	131/2 yr	131/2 yr
Second premolar	27 mo	28 mo	73/4 yr	71/2 yr	11 yr	111/4 yr	141/2 yr	15 yr
First molar	32 wk in utero	32 wk in utero	41/4 yr	33/4 yr	61/4 yr	6 yr	101/2 yr	101/2 yr
Second molar	27 mo	27 mo	73/4 yr	71/2 yr	121/2 yr	12 yr	153/4 yr	16 yr
Third molar	8 yr	9 yr	14 yr	14 yr	20 yr	20 yr	22 yr	22 yr

Table 2. Chronology of permanent tooth development mentioned by Proffit et al [12].

lateral incisors about a year later, and finally the maxillary laterals. There is a silent period of 1.5–2 years before the second active stage begins. This involves the exfoliation of deciduous canines and molars and replacement by permanent canines and premolars, together with the eruption of the second permanent molars. On the other hand, the third molars appear late in development stage. They usually start mineralization between 6 and 12 years, complete their crowns in 4 years and erupt and complete development during adolescence or early adulthood [12].

The total time taken for an individual tooth to develop is considerable, lasting from 2 to 3 years for the deciduous teeth and up to 8–12 years for the permanent teeth. In general, anterior permanent tooth crowns take 4–5 years and molar tooth crowns 3–4 years [16] and roots take approximately 6–7 years to grow. It has to be taken into consideration that the described general eruption sequence may change between individuals and genders. Tooth eruption is a complex process that can be influenced by several factors such as genetics, nutrition, preterm birth, gender differences, socioeconomic factors, craniofacial morphology, hormonal factors and various systemic diseases, which may cause earlier or delayed eruption [12]. Gender differences in the timing and duration of tooth formation are known, with dental maturity generally being more advanced in females than in males in permanent dentition in reverse of those for the deciduous dentition [17].

3. Dental age estimation methods

In literature, various methods are defined for dental age assessment that can be categorized as: visual, radiological, morphological, biochemical and histological methods [1, 18–21].

3.1. Visual method

Visual method is based on the evaluation of the sequence of teeth eruption in oral cavity and the morphological changes on tooth structure due to functions such as attrition, changes in color that are indicators of aging.

Fully formed teeth show aging changes. Thus, examination of dentition considering the tooth wear/attrition, tooth color and stains, periodontal status, etc. can provide valuable information on an individual's development and age [1, 18, 19, 21].

3.1.1. Evaluating tooth eruption

Tooth eruption in oral cavity follows a typical chronological pattern. As it was summarized in the above section, visual examination of the maxillary and mandibular dental arch may provide the dental age estimation up to 12–13 years of age in correspondence to the second molar eruption.

3.1.2. Tooth wear and attrition

Being a simple and convenient method, tooth wear is commonly used as a tool of individual's age estimation. Naturally, tooth wear increases with age. It is proportional to the time of exposure of teeth to the oral cavity [21]. This method does not need any invasive process such as tooth extraction or tissue preparation.

Tooth wear can be evaluated in conjunction to two different types of criteria: one is the area of tooth wear, which may be termed as a horizontal factor, and the second is the degree of dentin exposure, termed as a vertical factor. The combination of both horizontal and vertical factors should be considered to obtain a more accurate estimation of age [21, 22]. Hongwei and Jingtao [23] classified tooth wear scores into a 0- to 9-point scale based on the pattern, number and amount of tooth wear. Kim et al. [21] defined another simple and reliable scoring system, which can be applied to age estimation of individuals at any age ranges, as well (**Table 3**).

Tooth eruption being one of the visual methods in age estimation is considered to be not so reliable, as eruption is an ongoing process that includes inactive periods in a child's life when no tooth eruption occurs. It is also scarcely influenced by a number of local factors, such as the premature extraction of primary teeth causing a lack of space or the crowding of permanent teeth and systemic factors such as hereditary, functional, environmental, sexual, nutritional and metabolic factors [7, 24].

The secondary method, tooth wear, was defended to be an accurate method [23]; on the contrary, some authors advocated that tooth wear may not be reliable in age estimation [25]. As tooth wear is influenced by various factors that include functional (eating and chewing habits) or parafunctional habits, patterns of mandibular movement, bite force, saliva, diet, medication, diseases, geographical location, occupational and habitual environment and gender [21, 26].

Score	Premolar	Molar
0	**No visible wear**	
1	1P/1L	1P/1L/2P/2L
2	2P/2L/1S/1B	3P/3L/4P/4L/1S/1B/2S/2B
3	2S/2B	3S/3B/4S/4B
4	**Wear on more than 2/3 occlusal surface**	
5	1Pc/1Lc	1Pc/1Lc/2Pc/2Lc
6	2Pc/2Lc/1Sc/1Bc	3Pc/3Lc/4Pc/4Lc/1Sc/1Bc/2Sc/2Bc
7	2Sc/2Bc	3Sc/3Bc/4Sc/4Bc
8	**Concavity on more than 2/3 occlusal surface**	

Table 3. The Kim's scoring system of tooth wear [21]. P: point-like wear facet < ~1 mm. in diameter; L: linear wear facet < ~1 mm. in width; S: surface-like wear facet > ~1 mm. in diameter; B: band-like wear facet > ~1 mm. in width or wear facet involving more than two surfaces; c: concavity (wear of dentine). In the situation where a tooth has several different degrees of tooth wear, the highest degree should be selected as tooth wear score.

3.2. Radiographic methods

Dental age may be estimated by two approaches: based on the time of emergence of the tooth in the oral cavity and the pattern of tooth development, in another word the dental maturity stages. Dental maturity is considered to be more reliable than the emergence of teeth into the oral cavity with a high heritability and low coefficient variation, and to be independent of environmental effects, nutritional and endocrine status [6–8]. The development of each tooth can be assessed over long periods of time using radiographs in a continuous pattern, using different crown and root maturity stages of tooth formation as criteria [27, 28]. Radiological methods are based on the evaluation of tooth development on the various radiographic images as intraoral periapical, panoramic radiographs, digital and advanced imaging technologies to assess the extent of tooth mineralization from the moment when radiopaque spots become visible prior to tooth calcification until the tooth apex is closed (**Figure 1**) [10].

Beginning from the initial mineralization of a tooth, the crown formation, root growth, eruption of the tooth into the mouth and root apex maturation are assessed. Given that this method enables continuous evaluation of tooth development from birth until the completion of third molar teeth development [24, 29], it is mainly suitable for children-adolescents. It is also simple, a noninvasive and reproducible method that can be employed both on living and unknown dead.

The age determination on radiographs is based on the estimation of various features as follows:

1. Tooth germs appearance [14, 15, 30]
2. Beginning of mineralization both in the intrauterine life and after birth [14, 15, 30]
3. Amount of crown completion [14, 30, 31]
4. Eruption into the oral cavity [13–15, 30]
5. Degree of root completion of erupted or unerupted teeth [14, 15, 30]
6. Degree of resorption of deciduous teeth [14, 15]
7. Measurement of open apices [32, 33]
8. Volume of pulp chamber and root canals/formation of physiological secondary dentine [14, 34]
9. Tooth-to-pulp ratio [34, 35]
10. Third molar maturity [14, 15, 30, 34]

In children and adolescents, the chronological age estimation based on dental maturation is mainly done either by using the atlas approach or by using scoring systems. The dental development is divided into different stages that are assigned maturity scores for each tooth, evaluated through statistical analysis and then compared to known age standards in the "scoring method" [36].

3.2.1. *Atlas method*

The radiographic dental mineralization is compared with dental atlases that include a series of drawings with outlines of developing teeth and eruption relative to a corresponding age in the "Atlas method."

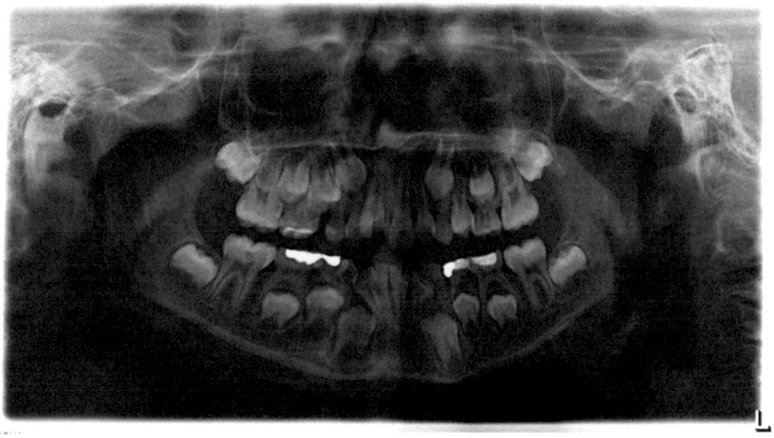

Figure 1. Panographic radiograph.

Kraus and Jordan [37] studied the early mineralization of teeth—deciduous teeth and the permanent first molar as well—in the intrauterine life. The development is described in 10 stages, expressed by Roman numerals from I to X; the IXth stage includes three stages and the Xth stage includes five stages [14]. Schour and Masseler [38, 39] studied the development of deciduous and permanent teeth, describing 21 chronological steps from 4 months to 21 years of age and published the numerical development charts for them without considering gender differences. Moorees et al. [40] evaluated the dental development in the 14 stages of mineralization ranging from 'cusp formation' to 'root apex closure' for developing single and multirooted permanent teeth by using panoramic or lateral oblique radiographs and the mean age for the corresponding stage was determined (**Figure 2**), taking into account the gender differences. Different tables are designed for each gender [41]. It provides an age estimate from 6 months up to the development of the third mandibular molar.

Later on, Anderson et al. [42] revised the method of Moorees et al. [40] by expanding the age range and comprehensive tables.

The London Atlas published by AlQahtani and colleagues [43] is a major improvement in estimating age compared to other dental charts and may be more practical than other dental atlases [44–46] with its high level of accuracy and repeatability. It provides an age estimate for individuals aged 28 weeks in utero to young individuals up to 23 years, so it enables the usage of the third molar. In addition, it can be used in cases where sex cannot be determined, as it provides sex-specific and sex-neutral dental charts [46]. Age is defined as the midpoint of an age category without an age range in the London Atlas. This could lead to a variation among investigators with the levels of education or experience.

3.2.2. Scoring method

Nolla [47] assessed the development of each tooth by evaluating the mineralization of permanent dentition in 10 stages. The radiograph of the patient is matched with a comparative figure and a total of the maxillary and mandibular teeth are assigned and the total is compared with

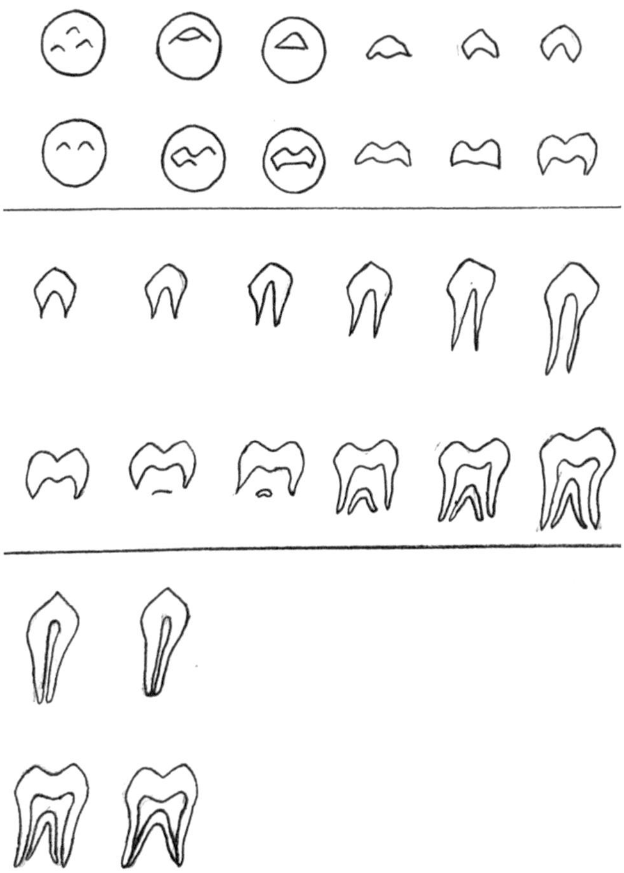

Figure 2. Schematic diagrams of the 14 dental development stages ranging from 'cusp formation' to 'root apex closure' defined by Moorees et al.

the table given by Nolla. The advantages of this method are that it can be applied to an individual with or without the third molar and that girls and boys are dealt with separately. Nolla's method allows the researcher to choose a stage from the 10 stages and also offers three inter-stage options for each stage. The increased number of stages may complicate the assessment and decrease accuracy of the method [48].

Different from Nolla's method instead of evaluating both maxillary and mandibular teeth, Demirjian et al. [49] determined only the dental maturity of the mandibular left seven permanent teeth (second molar to central incisors) based on eight tooth mineralization stages ("A" through "H") on a panoramic radiograph (**Figure 3**). The stages were allocated a biologically weighted score for each gender, and the sum of the scores provided an estimate of dental maturity, which was measured on a scale from 0 to 100 [49]. It was also reported to be reliable and reproducible [50].

Later, Demirjian and colleagues [51] developed three more methods, all of which are based on the analysis of the left mandibular dentition, but differ in relation to the type and/or number of

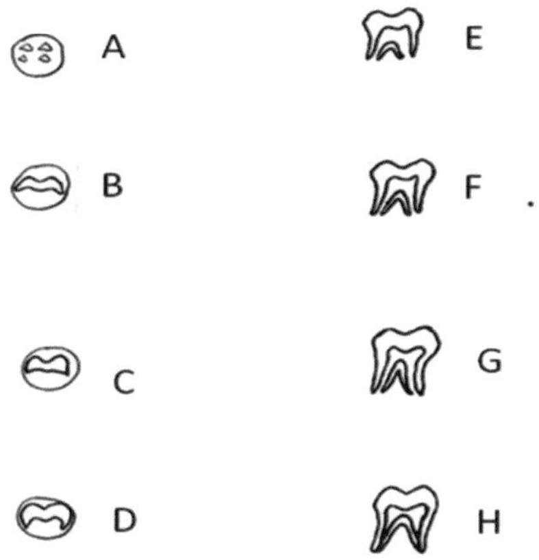

Figure 3. Schematic representation of the Demirjian, Goldstein and Tanner's stages: (A) in both uniradicular and multiradicular teeth, a beginning of calcification is seen at the superior level of the crypt in the form of an inverted cone or cones. There is no fusion of these calcification points; (B) fusion of calcified points forms one or more cusps, which unite to give a regularly outlined occlusal surface, or mineralized cusps are united so the mature coronal morphology is well defined; (C) crown half-formed, pulp chamber is evident, and dentinal deposition is occurring; (D) the crown formation is completed down to the cementoenamel junction (CEJ), pulp chamber has a trapezoidal form and beginning of root formation is seen; (E) initial formation of the radicular bifurcation is seen, and the root length is still less than the crown height; (F) the apex ends in a funnel shape; the root length is equal to or greater than the crown height; (G) the walls of the root canal are now parallel and its apical end is still partially open and (H) the apical end of the root canal is completely closed; the periodontal membrane has a uniform width around the root and the apex.

teeth used. These methods are as follows: 1. revised seven-tooth system [same teeth but with extended age ranges and two extra stages]; 2. four-teeth method [second molar (M2) to first premolar (PM1) inclusive]; and 3. Alternate four-teeth approach [the second incisive [12], first premolar [PM1], second premolar [PM2] and second molar [M2] [51, 52].

Although this method is reported to be simple, reliable and reproducible [50], it has some limitations as follows [30, 53, 54]:

1. This method excludes the subjects below the age of 4–4.5 years.
2. The evaluation cannot be applied in children lacking teeth.
3. This method may not express the retardation of dental development [excluding third molars] due to systemic diseases.
4. This method was developed based on the radiographic analysis of French-Canadian sub-adults; however, there may be a variation in the timing of dental development, both within and among the different populations in specific geographic regions [17, 55]. This may be attributed to different gene pools, differences in living conditions, climate, socioeconomic status, nutrition and secular changes [56–58] When the Demirjian data set was used for different populations, it mostly overestimated the age rather than underestimated it [59], which means that the subjects studied exhibited dentally advanced development compared with French-Canadian children [60]. Although some authors [29, 61] reject the applicability of the Demirjian standards in different populations, the others [62–65] support the applicability of these standards in particular age groups. Demirjian et al. [49] conjectured that the

scores for the stages would not vary much between populations, but the maturity standards may change appreciably.

The application of age estimation methods to populations that are dissimilar to the sample from which a particular method is derived is a critical issue in this field [46]. To overcome this drawback, the calculation of several 'modified' versions of the original Demirjian tables for different populations is offered [66–68]. The population-specific standards based on dental maturity curves are reported to be more accurate than the original curves [7, 24, 51, 69], but the variation among the geographical areas or different regions within the same country will still exist [70]. From another perspective, Liversidge et al. [62] mentioned that a positive secular trend during the last 25 years may partially explain the dental age overestimation by Demirjian's method recently found in different populations. In support, certain researchers have reported that dental development and age also follow secular trends and that teeth mature at an earlier chronological age than several decades ago [62, 71]. If the secular trend exists, correction of the reference standard that was developed using an affluent segment of more developed nations is significant for forensics, if the subject for which a dental age estimate is necessary is from a lower socioeconomic status in a developing country [72]. However, the other authors claimed that the level of tooth formation is not affected by secular trend, as it is predominantly determined by genetics, and less affected by environmental factors than other growth systems [73].

Willems [74] modified Demirjian's method based on a study on Belgian Caucasian population and formed new tables for the dental maturity for both genders by calculating chronological age based on the cumulative score of 4 teeth—first premolar, second premolar, first molar and second molar. This method is simpler and retains the advantage of Demirjian's method and there was a reduction in the overestimation of dental age. The estimated dental age is reported to be more accurate than Demirjian's method [75, 76].

Haavikko's method [77] is another method assessing the maturity of the teeth. Twelve radiographic stages—six relating to crown formation and six relating to root formation—of 4 permanent teeth are used to assess the dental age. This method is useful when any of the permanent teeth is missed.

As distinct from the methods evaluating the dental maturity, Cameriere et al. [33] measured open apices of the seven left permanent mandibular teeth in nonadults. They developed a linear regression formula for dental age estimation [46]. The following regression formula for age estimation is used

$$\text{Age} = 8.971 + 0.375\,\text{g} + 1.631 \times 5 + 0.674\,\text{N0} - 1.034\,\text{s} - 0.176\text{sN0} \quad (1)$$

where g is a variable equal to 1 for boys and 0 for girls, N0 is the number of teeth with apical ends of the root completely closed. The teeth with open apices are also considered. For teeth with one root, the distance between the inner sides of the open apex is measured, and for two roots, the sum of the distances between the inner sides of the two open apices is evaluated. To eliminate the magnification and angulation of the radiographs, the measurement of open apex is divided by the tooth length for each tooth. So, the measurements are normalized. Finally, s is the sum of the normalized open apices of the seven left permanent mandibular teeth.

In childhood and adolescent period, observing dentition maturity stages with radiographic method results in highly accurate age assessments. However, with increasing age, this method's accuracy will be weakened. The third molar is the only tooth with a tendency to continue developmental changes in late adolescence and early adulthood [5]. Third molar calcification stage is one of the few tools that can be used to assess age when development is nearing completion [8, 48, 50]. Many authors evaluated the third molar's maturity stages. Harris and Nortje [78] have given five stages of third molar root development in correspondence to the mean ages and mean length. Van Heerden [79] assessed the development of the mesial root of the third molar in five stages.

Clinically, the development of permanent dentition completes with the eruption of the third molar at the age of 17–21 years, after which the radiographic age estimation becomes difficult. However, this accuracy decreases as a person's dental development is completed. After that period, mature teeth cannot be used to estimate age because the time they completed developmental stages is unknown [48]. So that, other methods have to be used to estimate age by radiological determination. The reduction in size of the pulp cavity resulting from a secondary dentine deposition, which is proportional to the age of the individual, is one age predictor measurable in dental radiographs and tomographs as an alternative to more invasive methods [80–84]. In literature, two methods have been used:

1. Pulp-to-tooth ratio method by Kvaal [85]
2. Coronal pulp cavity index [86].

The coronal pulp cavity index [86] calculates the correlation between the reduction of the coronal pulp cavity and the chronological age. Only mandibular premolars and molars were considered on panoramic radiographs. The tooth-coronal index (TCI) is calculated for each tooth and regressed on the real age of the sample using the formula

$$\mathrm{TCI} = \mathrm{CPCH} \times 100/\mathrm{CL}. \tag{2}$$

where CPCH is the length of the coronal pulp cavity and CL is the length of the tooth crown.

Pulp-to-tooth ratio method: Kvall et al. calculated the pulp-tooth ratio for six mandibular and maxillary teeth, such as maxillary central and lateral incisors; maxillary second premolars; mandibular lateral incisor; mandibular canine and the first premolar (**Figure 4**). It is available to remove doubt as to whether a person is under 18 years of age and to calculate the age above this level. They measured pulp length and width as well as root length and width. Because of magnification and angulation on the radiographs, different ratios between root and pulp were measured.

The age is derived by using pulp-to-tooth ratios in the formula:

$$\mathrm{Age} = 129.8\text{–}[316.4 \times \mathrm{m}]\ [6.8 \times [\mathrm{W} - \mathrm{L}]]. \tag{3}$$

It has been reported that the pulp/tooth volume ratios in the cervical area were more correlated with age and that this correlation decreases toward the apex [87]. Also, the most marked reduction in volume ratio was observed between the second and the fifth decades of life in lower first and second premolars and between the second and the third decades of life in lower first premolars [87].

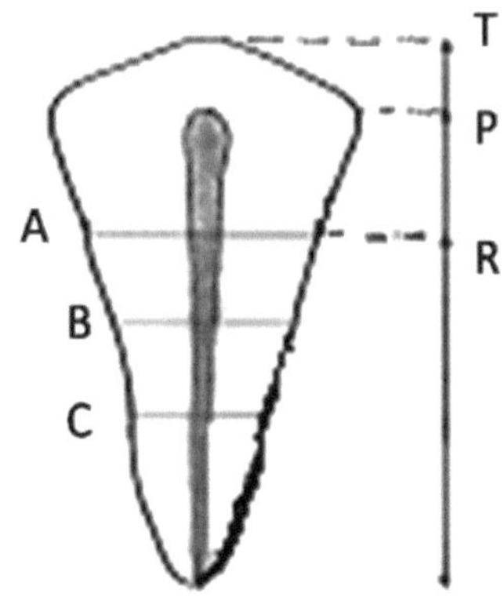

Figure 4. Dental measurements in Kvall's pulp-to-tooth ratio method: T, maximum tooth length; P, maximum pulp length; R, maximum root length; A, root and pulp width at cementoenamel junction; C, root and pulp width at mid-root level; B, root and pulp width halfway between levels A and C. Level A, the level of the cementoenamel junction (CEJ). Level B, midpoint between levels A and C. Level C, mid-root level between the CEJ and root apex.

This method is limited in finding the subjects retaining all the six teeth that were measured in this method. Also, there will be a certain amount of distortion when the curved arch of the jaws is projected on to a flat film. It would be better to use the parallel technique. Rotated teeth, teeth with enamel overlap, teeth with restorations, cavities, attrition and periapical pathological process cannot be used in this method, as well.

Using 3D images, the ratio of pulp/tooth volume can be calculated. Vandevoort et al. [34] reported a method using microfocused computed tomography on extracted teeth to compare pulp-to-tooth ratios in the determination of age. Yang et al. [80] used cone beam CT scanning and acquired the 3D images of teeth in living individuals.

In recent years, a software program named Dental Age Estimation® has been developed to automate the dental age calculations [88]. It includes the most accurate and often referenced morphological and radiological techniques that are reported in literature. The great advantage of the program is the immediate dental age estimation results. The borders of the pulp and tooth are automatically selected that minimizes the required time to obtain the area of tooth and pulp chamber, in addition, avoiding the calculating errors, the error associated with the observer, when performing the area selection reduces [89]. Also it enables the forensic odontologist to apply different techniques and provides a more reliable result.

Cameriere et al. [90] also developed the statistical regression model performed on digital radiographs by using upper canine pulp/tooth area ratio in adults. Given that, upper canines have certain advantages, such as their longer survival, less wear and the big size of the pulp chamber [91].

3.3. Morphological methods

Once dental development is complete, developmental stages could not be used for age estimation instead the indicators showing that dental structures undergo changes through life are being used. Morphological methods are based on assessment of ex-vivo teeth for age estimation of adults. The samples of the extracted tooth can be sectioned or unsectioned and observed with the eye or with microscope [1]. However, these methods may not be acceptable due to ethical, religious, cultural or scientific reasons.

In literature, many morphological methods are encountered. Gustafson [92], Dalitz [93], Bang and Ramm [94], Johanson [2], Maples [95] and Solheim [96] developed various morphological methods.

The first technique was published by *Gustafson* in 1950 [92]. Gustafson [92] and Thoma [97] described the morphological changes occurring in the dental tissues by increasing age and noted the following changes:

a. Attrition of the incisal or occlusal surfaces due to mastication [A]

b. Periodontitis [P]—the loss of periodontal attachment

c. Secondary dentin [S]—the amount of coronal secondary dentine formation

d. Cementum apposition [C] at the root apex

e. Root resorption [R] amount

f. Transparency of the root [T]

Each criterion was ranked and allotted 0, 1, 2 and 3 points. The score values of each age change are added according to the following formula:

$$\mathrm{A_n} + \mathrm{P_n} + \mathrm{S_n} + \mathrm{C_n} + \mathrm{R_n} + \mathrm{T_n} = x(\text{overall score}). \tag{4}$$

The exact equation calculated was: y (age) = 11.43 + 4.56x.

This method cannot be used in a living person, only in dead when extraction of a tooth is allowed [96]. It is a subjective method [94] and time-consuming [95]. Periodontitis is often impossible to determine due to the decomposition of a soft tissue [95]. It neglects the possible interrelationships among the criteria [94] and population differences in diet habits with a resultant effect of attrition on tooth.

Dalitz [93] revised Gustafson's method and suggested a 5-point system from 0 to 4, rather than 4-point system to obtain a greater accuracy with the suggested formula. He mentioned that root resorption and secondary cementum formation could be disregarded.

$$\mathrm{E} = 8.691 + 5.146\mathrm{A} + 5.338\mathrm{P} + 1.866\mathrm{S} + 8.411\ \mathrm{T}. \tag{5}$$

In this method, 12 anterior teeth are evaluated; bicuspids and molar teeth are not taken into account.

Johanson [2] evaluated for the same six criteria of Gustafson's method in seven different stages with corresponding scores from 0 to 3. Johanson made a more detailed study of the root transparency and stated that it is more clear when the thickness of the ground section of the tooth was 0.25 mm.

The following formula was recommended:

$$\text{Age} = 11.02 + [5.14 \times A] + [2.3 \times S] + [4.14 \times P] + [3.71 \times C] + [5.57 \times R] + [8.98 \times T]. \quad (6)$$

Where A is attrition, S is secondary dentine formation, P is periodontal attachment loss, C is cement apposition, R is root resorption and T is apical translucent [Q].

Solheim [96] reported another method by using five of the criteria of Gustafson's method [attrition, secondary dentin, periodontitis, cementum apposition and root transparency] in addition to another three new criteria: the surface roughness, color and sex. He recommended not using this method on mandibular canines and second premolars because of the weakest relationship between the parameters and age on these teeth. Two set of formulas were presented: one including sex and color and the other without them, because these factors were not always determinable in deceased individuals. The color may be differentiated due to changes or reactions to the environment and compared with teeth from living individuals; teeth removed from deceased bodies were darker.

Bang and Ramm [94] presented a simple and accurate method for age estimation based on the measurement of only one criterion: the length of the apical translucent zone of only incisors and cuspids (**Figure 5**).

For translucent zones ≤9 mm., a formula Age = $B_0 + (B_1 \times X) + (B_2 \times X^2)$ is used, and if translucent zones > 9 mm., another formula is used: Age = $B_0 + (B_1 \times X)$ [Q].

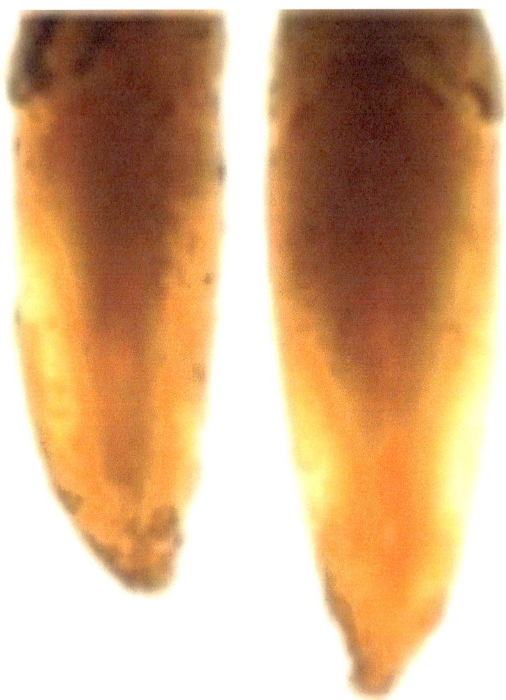

Figure 5. Apical translucent zone.

The authors mentioned that transparency of the root dentin advances during the third decade starting at the tip of the root and extending coronally with age. The teeth were sectioned. The length of the root was measured buccally from the cementoenamel junction to the apex. The transparent root dentin was measured midway between the pulp chamber and the root periphery where the translucent/opaque boundary across the root is fairly horizontal. With this method, good results are obtained by measuring intact roots only. The method is simple, objective and rather fast compared to other methods and can be applied without extensive training or expensive equipment. However, it was difficult to make accurate measurements in molars and bicuspids [94].

Similar to Bang and Ramm [94], Lamendin [98, 99] emphasized that root translucency was the most important one in Gustafson's seven aging criteria. Differently, not only the translucency but also the periodontal tissue level is determined as well. And the measurements are made only on the entire extracted single rooted tooth—the incisors or canines—without any preparation. In their method, the age in years at death is obtained by the following formula:

$$\text{Age} = \left[\left[\text{Periodontosis}/\text{root length} \times 0.18\right] + \left[\text{translucency}/\text{root length} \times 0.42\right]\right] \times 100 + 25.53. \quad (7)$$

where root length is the distance between the apex of the root and at the cementoenamel junction; *periodontosis* is the distance between the crown and soft tissue attachment line; *translucency* is evaluated by looking at the tooth exposed to a light box and the length of the transparent zone at the apex of the root is measured. This method is simple and differences between observers are low. However, it is not suitable in young adults as the translucency due to the deposition of hydroxyapatite crystals in the dental tubuli begins after the age of 25. In addition, it gives unreliable age estimation on elder subjects with periodontal disease. The major adversity of this method is the absence of single root tooth that is frequently seen in the elderly or disturbed skeletal remains. Also, it has to be taken into consideration that if there is a long postmortem interval [at least decades] the translucency of the root might be affected by taphonomic factors.

Maples [95] also modified Gustafson's method by using only two criteria of the total six Gustafson recommended: secondary dentine formation and root transparency. With this method, researcher error is expected to be lessened. Teeth with broken crowns, lost cementum and periodontal attachment may still give accurate age estimates. As it does not evaluate the attrition, the bias due to the dietary differences is expected to be decreased [41].

3.4. Biochemical methods

In prenatal stage, up to 6 months, radiological methods cannot be accurate in dental age estimation given that the dentin and enamel images are radiolucent. Therefore, *Stack's method* [100] is suitable to overcome this restriction. It was demonstrated that the dry weight of the mineralized tooth cusps gives an approximate age of the child by using gravimetric methods. Fetal age is linearly related to the square root of the weight of mineralized tissue in the deciduous anterior teeth during the last trimester. At 6 months intrauterine life, the weight is 60 mg; in the newborn child, the teeth weigh 0.5 g, which increases to 1.8 g after 6 months.

Deutsch et al. [101] reported that both the weight and crown height of the anterior teeth were correlated with fetal age as well.

In adults, following completion of the growth period, age estimation by radiological methods becomes not sufficiently accurate [10, 102]. Alternative methods such as biochemical and histological methods are preferred in adults.

The biochemical methods determine alterations in ion levels with age. For instance, the calcium/phosphorus ratio in peritubular dentine increases significantly with age and the rate of racemization of D and L enantiomers of aspartic acid residues in the collagen of dentin is time-dependent [103].

In literature, aspartic acid racemization [104, 105] has been studied for the aim of developing age estimation standards in adults. Although aspartic acid racemization is affected by environmental factors, such that with increasing temperature, racemization increases also, it is demonstrated to be an accurate age estimation method [106]. However, the mentioned method is invasive and expensive and also requires specialized equipment and expertise [104, 105]. In addition, it is not suitable in living individuals [107].

The biochemical methods are based on the racemization of amino acids. The racemization of amino acids is a reversible first-order reaction and is relatively rapid in living tissues in which metabolism is slow. Aspartic acid has been reported to have the highest racemization rate of all amino acids and to be stored during aging. In particular, L-aspartic acids are converted into D-aspartic acids, and so, the levels of D-aspartic acid in human enamel, dentine and cementum increase with age. The D/L ratio has been shown to be highly correlated with age [108]. Helfman and Bada [109] reported studies that focused on the racemization of amino acids and obtained a significant correlation between age and ratio of D/L enantiomers in aspartic acid in enamel and coronal dentin.

The racemization rate of the cementum shows the fastest reaction than enamel and dentine.

On the other hand, dentine showed the highest correlation with actual age [108]. With this method, age determination is not suitable with extensive crown destruction in postmortem examination [110] rather than the extraction of the teeth. Ritz et al. [110] suggested another less invasive way of racemization estimation by dentinal biopsy specimens taken from molars in living subjects. The extension of aspartic acid racemization is higher in deep layers, so biopsy layer had a noteworthy influence. The cavities are then treated with filling materials.

3.5. Histological method

Histological methods require the preparation of the tissues for detailed microscopic examination. This technique is more appropriate for postmortem situations. In prenatal stage, up to 6 months, the dentin and the enamel images are not radiopaque enough to be visualized on radiographs. The histological methods can detect mineralization before being detected in the radiographs. Prenatal dental maturity can be assessed by using dissection and alizarin staining of fetal tooth germs [9]. Initiation of mineralization, as visualized by alizarin staining, takes place in the first permanent molars between 28 and 32 fetal weeks with the mandibular germs being slightly in advance than those of the maxilla [9].

The estimation period of survival of an infant in perinatal period using *neonatal line* as a line of reference can give the exact age of the baby in days [111]. The neonatal lines, present in both enamel and dentin of the permanent teeth, are an optical phenomenon produced due to alteration in the dimension, degree and mineralization of enamel prisms caused due to the sudden change from intrauterine to extrauterine environment [112]. Observing the neonatal lines can be used for assessing the amount of pre- and postnatal enamel formation. In primary enamel, the rate of enamel formation is 2.5–4.5 μ/day [113]. Cross striations are seen across enamel rods representing the daily incremental deposition of enamel [114], and this can be used to find the exact age of the baby in days by counting the cross striations from the neonatal line [111]. Neonatal lines can be used to differentiate between live birth and still birth and are an important tool in forensic cases and for preepidemiological studies. However, the absence of the neonatal line is not always an indicator of still birth [30]. The main limitation of using neonatal line for estimation is that a couple of days of survival is necessary for the neonatal line to develop. Besides, the detection of neonatal line depends on various factors like axis of tooth section, thickness of the section and light source used.

Cementum annulations indeed are a reflection of age, as well. The incremental lines in the tooth cementum can be used as a marker more reliable than any other morphological or histological traits in the human skeleton [4, 51]. A method for preparing human teeth for evaluation involving collection, identification, measuring, sectioning, cleaning, acid etching, staining and mounting is reported. Sections of 100-pm thick are stained with cresyl fast violet as a stain of choice and are photographed using standard light microscopic techniques, as well as, Nomarski interference microscopy. Acellular cementum bands viewed in transmitted polarized light are characterized by alternating parallel opaque and translucent wider bands. Countability of annulations from photographic enlargements was evaluated. However, it is not always easy to count [115]. Miller et al. [116] reported that determining chronologic age in humans from cementum annulations is not possible.

While using all these methods, the following has to be taken into consideration:

- Gender differences may exist. Tooth wear scores in males are found to be higher than those in females. Males show better development of masticatory muscles than females. Thus, males could exert a stronger bite force than females [21]. Also sexual dimorphism is indicated in the timing and duration of tooth formation, with dental maturity generally being more advanced in females than in males in permanent dentition in reverse of those for the deciduous dentition [17]. If only pulp volume is measured and used as age indicator, there is a significant difference between the accuracy for males and females [117, 118]. To account for this, many dental age estimation methods publish sex-specific formulae or charts. While sex-specific formulae or charts increase accuracy, depending on the condition of the remains, it may be impossible to confidently determine the sex of nonadults without the use of DNA, which may or may not be present [46]. When sex is unknown, the most accurate method is Willems followed by Demirjian and then Haavikko first premolar [76]. Additionally, sex has no statistically significant effect on age estimation, when pulp-to-tooth ratio is calculated [117, 118].
- There are controversial results in the effect of orthodontic treatment on age estimation [119, 120]. Orthodontic treatment may cause external root resorption with subsequent root

shortening and reduction in pulp chamber dimensions, owing to secondary dentine formation. This may cause a potential risk of overestimation while using the methods based on secondary dentine formation and the variation of pulp/tooth dimensions with age. If that were to be the case, it would be necessary to develop specific standards for orthodontically treated participants. Contrarily, it was reported that the changes caused by orthodontic treatment do not have any significant effect on age estimation when Kvaal et al.'s method is applied [121].

- There may be a significant delay in dental age in the subjects with dental agenesis.

4. Conclusion

Chronologic age estimation from teeth for the postmortem evaluation is well established. In this chapter, the different techniques and considered studies were overviewed in conjunction with their advantages and disadvantages. It needs to be taken into consideration that rather than restricting on one age estimation technique, using the other available techniques additionally and performing repetitive measurements may be beneficial for accurate age estimation.

In lights of previous studies, the following can be concluded:

- In prenatal stage, up to 6 months, the dentin and the enamel images are not radiopaque enough to be visualized on radiographs. In that period, the usage of gravimetric method and alizarin staining of fetal tooth germs are recommended in the age assessment.
- In children and adolescents, the radiographic methods that are based on the evaluation of tooth development to assess the extent of tooth mineralization are preferred.
- Third molar calcification stage is one of the few tools that can be used to assess age when development is nearing completion. Clinically, the development of permanent dentition completes with the eruption of the third molar at the age of 17–21 years, after which the radiographic age estimation becomes difficult.
- After the apex closure of third molar, the coronal pulp cavity index or pulp-to-tooth ratio method is used.
- Once dental development is complete, the invasive morphological and histological methods are preferred. Gustafson morphological method is the most accurate around 40–50 years and with increasing inaccuracy in younger and especially in older age groups. Biochemical age determination procedures based on aspartic acid racemization in dentin is more reliable; however, an influence of iatrogenic and carious lesions on the composition of the surrounding dentin and thus on aspartic acid racemization cannot be excluded.
- Dental maturation of children at similar ages in different ethnic groups may differ due to different gene pools, living conditions, climate, socioeconomic status, nutrition and secular changes, which may affect the accuracy of the dental age estimation. To overcome this limitation, population-specific standards based on dental maturity curves can be used.

- An alternate imaging modality is the CT scanning to acquire 3-dimensional images of teeth. It is found to be a more reliable technology for use in dental age estimation.
- The software programs enable the forensic odontologist to apply different techniques, provide a more reliable and immediate result, and avoid calculation errors.

Author details

Fatma Deniz Uzuner*, Emine Kaygısız and Nilüfer Darendeliler

*Address all correspondence to: fduzuner@yahoo.com.tr

Faculty of Dentistry, Department of Orthodontics, Gazi University, Ankara, Turkey

References

[1] Willems G, Moulin-Romsee C, Solheim T. Non-destructive dental-age calculation methods in adults: Intra- and inter-observer effects. Forensic Science International. 2002;**126**:221-226. DOI: 10.1016/S0379-0738(02)00081-6

[2] Johanson G. Age determination from human teeth. Odontologisk Revy Supplement. 1971;**22**:1-126

[3] Reesu GV, Augustine J, Urs AB. Forensic considerations when dealing with incinerated human dental remains. Journal of Forensic and Legal Medicine. 2015;**29**:13-17. DOI: 10.1016/j.jflm.2014.10.006

[4] Nayar AK, Parhar S, Thind G, Sharma A, Sharma D. Determination of age, sex, and blood group from a single tooth. Journal of Forensic Dental Sciences. 2017;**9**:10-14

[5] Lewis JM, Senn DR. Dental age estimation utilizing third molar development: A review of principles, methods, and population studies used in the United States. Forensic Science International. 2010;**20**:79-83. DOI: 10.1016/j.forsciint.2010.04.042

[6] McKenna CJ, James H, Taylor JA, Townsend GC. Tooth development standards for South Australia. Australian Dental Journal. 2002;**47**:223-227. DOI: 10.1111/j.1834-7819.2002.tb00333.x

[7] Celik S, Zeren C, Çelikel A, Yengil E, Altan A. Applicability of the Demirjian method for dental assessment of southern Turkish children. Journal of Forensic and Legal Medicine. 2014;**25**:1-5. DOI: 10.1016/j.jflm.2014.04.006

[8] Sisman Y, Uysal T, Yagmur F, Ramoglu SI. Third-molar evelopment in relation to chronologic age in Turkishchildren and young adults. The Angle Orthodontist. 2007;**77**:1040-1045. DOI: 10.2319/101906-430.1

[9] Cunningham C, Scheuer L, Black S. Developmental Juvenile Osteology. 2nd ed. San Diego: Wiley; 2016. DOI: 10.1046/j.1469-7580.2001.199303692.x

[10] Kotecha SD. Dental age estimation in children: A review. Forensic Research Criminology International Journal. 2016;**3**:00085. DOI: 10.15406/frcij.2016.03.00085

[11] Stavrianos C, Mastagas D, Stavrianou I, Karaiskou O. Dental age estimation of adults: A review of methods and principals. Research Journal of Medical Sciences. 2008;**2**:258-268. DOI: rjmsci.2008.258.268

[12] Proffit W, Fields HW, Sarver DM. Contemporary Orthodontics. 5th ed. St. Louis: Mosby; 2012. pp. 66-88

[13] Masthan KMK. Age estimation by teeth. In: Textbook of Forensic Odontology. New Delhi: Jaypee Brothers Medical Publishers [P] Ltd; 2009. pp. 92-97

[14] Masthan KMK. Age and sex. In: Textbook of Forensic Odontology. New Delhi: Jaypee Brothers Medical Publishers [P] Ltd; 2009. pp. 59-65

[15] Whittakar DK, McDonald DG. Age Determination from Teeth. A Color Atlas of Forensic Dentistry. England: Wolfe Medical Publications Ltd; 1989. pp. 58-66

[16] Reid DJ, Dean MC. Variation in modern human enamel formation times. Journal of Human Evolution. 2006;**50**:329-346

[17] Mincer HH, Harris EF, Berryman HE. The A.B.F.O. study of third molar development and its use as an estimator of chronological age. Journal of Forensic Sciences. 1993;**38**:379-390. DOI: 10.1520/JFS13418J

[18] Kvaal S. Collection of post mortem data: DVI protocols and quality assurance. Forensic Science International. 2006;**159**:12-14. DOI: 10.1016/j.forsciint.2006.02.003

[19] Reppien K, Sejrsen B, Lynnerup N. Evaluation of post-mortem estimated dental age versus real age: A retrospective 21-year survey. Forensic Science International. 2006;**159**(Suppl 1): S84-S88. DOI: 10.1016/j.forsciint.2006.02.021

[20] Seligrnan DA, Pullinger AG, Solberg WK. The prevalence of dental attrition and its association with factors of age, gender, occlusion, and TMJ syrnptomatology. Journal of Dental Research. 1988;**67**:1323-1333. DOI: 10.1177/00220345880670101601

[21] Kim YK, Kho HS, Lee KH. Age estimation by cclusal tooth wear. Journal of Forensic Sciences. 2000;**45**:303-309. DOI: 10.1520/JFS14683J

[22] Kambe T, Yonernitsu K, Kibayashi K, Tsunenari S. Application of a computer assisted image analyzer to the assessment of area and number of sites of dental attrition and its use for age estimation. Forensic Science International. 1991;**50**:97-109. DOI: 10.1016/0379-0738(91)90138-9

[23] Hongwei S, Jingtao J. The estimation of tooth age from attrjtion of the occlusal surface. Medicine, Science, and the Law. 1989;**29**:69-73

[24] Erdem AP, Yamac E, Erdem MA, Sepet E, Aytepe Z. A new method to estimate dental age. Acta Odontologica Scandinavica. 2013;**71**:590-598. DOI: 10.3109/00016357.2012.700062

[25] Gustafson G. Forensic Odontology. 1st ed. London: Elsevier; 1966. pp. 103-139

[26] Dahl BL, Carlsson GE, Ekfeldt A. Occlusal wear of teeth and restorative materials. A review of classification, etiology, mechanisms of wear, and some aspects of restorative procedures. Acta Odontologica Scandinavica. 1993;**51**:299-311. DOI: 10.3109/00016359309040581

[27] Liversidge HM, Smith BH, Maber M. Bias and accuracy of age estimation using developing teeth in 946 children. American Journal of Physical Anthropology. 2010;**143**:545-554. DOI: 10.1002/ajpa.21349

[28] Mani SA, Naing L, John J, Samsudin AR. Comparison of two methods of dental age estimation in 7-15-year-old Malays. International Journal of Paediatric Dentistry. 2008;**18**:380-388. DOI: 10.1111/j.1365-263X.2007.00890.x

[29] Hegde RJ, Sood PB. Dental maturity as an indicator of chronological age: Radiographic evaluation of denatl age in 6-13 years children of Belgaum using Demirjian methods. Journal of the Indian Society of Pedodontics and Preventive Dentistry. 2002;**20**:132-138

[30] Ciapparelli L. The chronology of dental development and age assessment. In: Clark DH, editor. Practical Forensic Odontology. 1st ed. Oxford: Butterworth-Heinmann Ltd; 1992. pp. 20-42

[31] Cameriere R, Ferrante L, Belcastro M, Bonfiaglioli B, Rastelli E, et al. Age estimation by pulp/tooth ratio in canines by periapical X-rays. Journal of Forensic Sciences. 2007;**52**:166-170. DOI: 10.1111/j.1556-4029.2007.00530.x

[32] Cameriere R, Ferrante L, Cingoloni M. Age estimation in children by measurement of open apices in teeth. International Journal of Legal Medicine. 2006;**120**:49-52. DOI: 10.1007/s00414-005-0047-9

[33] Rai B, Anand SC. Age estimation in children from dental radiograph: A regression equation. The Internet Journal of Biological Anthropology. 2008;**1**:1-5

[34] Vandevoort FM, Bergamans L, Cleyenbreugel JV, Bielen DJ, Lambrechts P, Wevers M. Age calculation using X-ray microfocus computed tomographical scanning of teeth: A pilot study. Journal of Forensic Sciences. 2004;**49**:787-790. DOI: 10.1520/JFS2004069

[35] Singaraju S, Sharda P. Age estimation using pulp-tooth area ratio: A digital image analysis. Journal of Forensic Dental Sciences. 2009;**1**:37-41. DOI: 10.4103/0974-2948.50888

[36] Sweet D. Why a dentist for identification. Forensic odontology. Dental Clinics of North America. 2001;**45**:217-249

[37] Kraus BS, Jordan RE. The Human Dentition before Birth. Philadelphia: Lea and Febiger; 1965. 218 p

[38] Schour I, Massler M. Development of human dentition. Journal of the American Dental Association (1939). 1941;**20**:379-427

[39] Schour I, Massler M. Studies in tooth development: The growth pattern of human teeth. Journal of the American Dental Association (1939). 1940;**27**:1778-1793

[40] Moorees CFA, Fanning EA, Hunt EE. Age variation of formation stages for ten permanent teeth. Journal of Dental Research. 1963;**42**:1490-1502. DOI: 10.1177/00220345630420062701

[41] Anderson DL, Thompson GW, Popovitch F. Age of attainment of minerilization stages of the permanent dentition. Journal of Forensic Sciences. 1976;**21**:191-200. DOI: 10.1520/JFS10353J

[42] Willems G. A review of the most commonly used dental age estimation techniques. The Journal of Forensic Odonto-Stomatology. 2001;**19**:9-17

[43] AlQahtani SJ, Hector MP, Liversidge HM. Brief communication: The London atlas of human tooth development and eruption. American Journal of Physical Anthropology. 2010;**142**:481-490. DOI: 10.1002/ajpa.21258

[44] Schour I, Massler M. The development of the human dentition. Journal of the American Dental Association (1939). 1941;**28**:1153-1160

[45] Ubelaker DH. Human Skeletal Remains: Excavation, Analysis, Interpretation. 1st ed. Chicago, IL: Taraxacum; 1978

[46] Santana SA, Bethard JD, Moore TL. Accuracy of dental age in nonadults: A comparison of TwoMethods for age estimation using radiographs of developing teeth. Journal of Forensic Sciences. 2017;**62**:1320-1325. DOI: 10.1111/1556-4029.13434

[47] Nolla CM. The development of permanent teeth. Journal of Dentistry for Children. 1960;**27**:253-266

[48] Kırzıoğlu Z, Ceyhan D. Accuracy of different dental age estimation methods on Turkish children. Forensic Science International. 2012;**216**:61-67. DOI: 10.1016/j.forsciint.2011.08.018

[49] Demirjian A, Goldstein H, Tanner JM. A new system of dental age assessment. Human Biology. 1973;**45**:211-227

[50] Kaygısız E, Uzuner FD, Yeniay A, Darendeliler N. Secular trend in the maturation of permanent teeth in a sample of Turkish children over the past 30 years. Forensic Science International. 2016;**259**:155-160. DOI: 10.1016/j.forsciint.2015.12.031

[51] Flood SJ, Franklin D, Turlach BA, MGJ. A comparison of Demirjian's four dental development methods for forensic age estimation in South Australian sub-adults. Journal of Forensic and Legal Medicine. 2013;**20**:875-883. DOI: 10.1016/j.jflm.2013.07.002

[52] Demirjian A, Goldstein H. New systems for dental maturity based on seven and four teeth. Annals of Human Biology. 1976;**3**:411-421

[53] Babar MG, Iqbal S, Jan A. Essential guidelines for forensic dentistry. Pakistan Oral & Dental Journal. 2008;**27**:79-84

[54] Ardakani F, Bashardoust N, Sheikhha M. The accuracy of dental panoramic radiography as an indicator of chronological age in Iranian individuals. The Journal of Forensic Odonto-Stomatology. 2007;**25**:30-35

[55] Al-Tuwirqi A, Holcombe T, Seow WK. A study of dental development in a Caucasian population compared with a non-caucasian population. European Archives of Paediatric Dentistry. 2011;**12**:26-30

[56] Cantekin K, Sekerci AE, Peduk K, Delikan E, Ozakar Ilday N, Demirbuga S, Miloglu O. Dental age assessment for different climatic regions. The American Journal of Forensic Medicine and Pathology. 2014;**35**:197-200. DOI: 10.1097/PAF.0000000000000096

[57] Heuze Y, Cardoso HF. Testing the quality of nonadult Bayesian dental age assessment methods to juvenile skeletal remains: The Lisbon collection children and secular trend effects. American Journal of Physical Anthropology. 2008;**135**:275-283. DOI: 10.1002/ajpa.20741

[58] Pelsmaekers B, Loos R, Carels C, Derom C, Vlietinck R. The genetic contribution to dental maturation. Journal of Dental Research. 1997;**76**:1337-1340. DOI: 10.1177/00220345970760070201

[59] Sasso A, Spalj S, Mady Maričić B, Sasso A, Cabov T, Legović M. Secular trend in the development of permanent teeth in a population of Istria and the Littoral region of Croatia. Journal of Forensic Sciences. 2013;**58**:673-677. DOI: 10.1111/j.1556-4029.2012.02301.x

[60] Jayaraman J, Wong HM, King NM, Roberts GJ. The French-Canadian data set of Demirjian for dental age estimation: A systematic review and meta-analysis. Journal of Forensic and Legal Medicine. 2013;**20**:373-381. DOI: 10.1016/j.jflm.2013.03.015

[61] Bagherpour A, Imanimoghaddam M, Bagherpour MR, Einolghozati M. Dental age assessment among Iranian children aged 6–13 years using the Demirjian method. Forensic Science International. 2010;**197**:121.e1-121.e4. DOI: 10.1016/j.forsciint.2009.12.051

[62] Liversidge HM, Speechly T, Hector MP. Dental maturation in British children: Are Demirjian's standards applicable? International Journal of Paediatric Dentistry. 1999; **9**(4):263-269

[63] Nik-Hussein NN, Kee KM, Gan P. Validity of Demirjian and Willems methods for dental age estimation for Malaysian children aged 5–15 years old. Forensic Science International. 2011;**204**:208.e1-208.e6. DOI: 10.1016/j.forsciint.2010.08.020

[64] Cruz-Landeira A, Linares-Argote J, Martínez-Rodríguez M, Rodríguez-Calvo MS, Otero XL, Concheiro L. Dental age estimation in Spanish and Venezuelan children. Comparison of Demirjian and Chaillet's scores. International Journal of Legal Medicine. 2010;**124**(2):105-112. DOI: 10.1007/s00414-009-0380-5

[65] Tunc ES, Koyuturk AE. Dental age assessment using Demirjian's method on northern Turkish children. Forensic Science International. 2008;**175**:23-26. DOI: 10.1016/j.forsciint.2007.04.228

[66] Chaillet N, Willems G, Demirjian A. Dental maturity in Belgian children using Demirjian's method and polynomial functions: new standard curves for forensic and clinical use. Journal of Forensic Odonto-Stomatology. 2004;**22**(2):18-27

[67] Leurs IH, Wattel E, Aartman IH, Etty E, Prahl-Andersen B. Dental age in Dutch children. European Journal of Orthodontics. 2005;**27**:309-314. DOI: 10.1093/ejo/cji010

[68] Chaillet N, Nyström M, Kataja M, Demirjian A. Dental maturity curves in Finnish children: Demirjian's method revisited and polynomial functions for age estimation. Journal of Forensic Sciences. 2004;**49**(6):1324-1331

[69] Sarkar S, Kailasam S, Mahesh KP. Accuracy of estimation of dental age in comparison with chronological age in Indian population—A comparative analysis of two formulas. Journal of Forensic and Legal Medicine. 2013;**20**:230-233. DOI: 10.1016/j.jflm.2012.09.007

[70] Baghdadi ZD, Pani SC. Accuracy of population-specific Demirjian curves in the estimation of dental age of Saudi children. International Journal of Paediatric Dentistry. 2012;**22**:125-131. DOI: 10.1111/j.1365-263X.2011.01179.x

[71] Krailassiri S, Anuwongnukroh N, Dechkunakorn S. Relationships between dental calcification stages and skeletal maturity indicators in Thai individuals. The Angle Orthodontist. 2002;**72**:155-166. DOI: 10.1043/0003-3219(2002)072<0155:RBDCSA>2.0.CO;2

[72] Sasso A, Legovic M, Mady Maricic B, Pavlic A, Spalj S. Secular trend of earlier onset and decelerated development of third molars: Evidence from Croatia. Forensic Science International. 2015;**249**:202-206. DOI: 10.1016/j.forsciint.2015.02.002

[73] Parner ET, Heidmann JM, Vaeth M, Poulsen S. A longitudinal study of time trends in the eruption of permanent teeth in Danish children. Archives of Oral Biology. 2001;**46**:425-431. DOI: 10.1016/S0003-9969(01)00002-4

[74] Willems G, Van Olmen A, Spiessens B, Carels C. Dental age estimation in Belgian children: Demirjian's technique revistited. Journal of Forensic Sciences. 2001;**46**:893-895. DOI: 10.1520/JFS15064J

[75] Maber M, Liversidge HM, Hector MO. Accuracy of age estimation of radiographic methods using developing teeth. Forensic Science International. 2006;**159**:S68-S73. DOI: 10.1016/j.forsciint.2006.02.019

[76] Phillips VM, van Wyk Kotze TJ. Testing standard methods of dental age estimation by moorrees, fanning and hunt and demirjian, goldstein and tanner on three south african children samples. Journal of Forensic Odonto-Stomatology. 2009;**27**(2):20-28

[77] Haavikko K. Tooth formation age estimated on a few selected teeth—A simple method for clinical use. Proceedings of the Finnish Dental Society. 1974;**70**:15-19

[78] Harris MJ, Nortjé CJ. The mesial root of the third mandibular molar. A possible indicator of age. The Journal of Forensic Odonto-Stomatology. 1984;**2**:39-43

[79] Van Heerden PJ. The Mesial Root of the Third Mandibular Molar as a Possible Indicator of Age. Dissertation for Diploma in Forensic Odontology. London Hospital Medical College; 1985.

[80] Yang F, Jacobs R, Willems G. Dental age estimation through volume matching of teeth imaged by cone-beam CT. Forensic Science International. 2006;**15**(159 Suppl 1):S78-S83. DOI: 10.1016/j.forsciint.2006.02.031

[81] Vodanović M, Dumančić J, Galić I, Savić Pavičin I, Petrovečki M, Cameriere R, Brkić H. Age estimation in archaeological skeletal remains: Evaluation of four non-destructive age calculation methods. The Journal of Forensic Odonto-Stomatology. 2011;**29**:14-21

[82] Fabbri PF, Viva S, Ferrante L, Lonoce N, Tiberi I, Cameriere R. Radiological tooth/pulp ratio in canines and individual age estimation in a sample of adult neolithic skeletons from Italy. American Journal of Physical Anthropology. 2015;**158**:423-430. DOI: 10.1002/ajpa.22796

[83] De Angelis D, Gibelli D, Fabbri P, Cattaneo C. Dental age estimation helps create a new identity. The American Journal of Forensic Medicine and Pathology. 2015;**36**(3):219-220. DOI: 10.1097/PAF.0000000000000178

[84] Kvall SI, Solheim T. A non-destructive dental method for age estimation. Journal of Forensic Odonto-Stomatology. 1994;**12**:6-11

[85] Kvaal SI, Kolltveit KM, Thomsen IO, Solheim T. Age estimation of adults from dental radiographs. Forensic Science International. 1995;**74**:175-185

[86] Panchbhai AS. Dental radiographic indicators, a key to age estimation. Dento Maxillo Facial Radiology. 2011;**40**:199-212. DOI: 10.1259/dmfr/19478385

[87] Aboshi H, Takahashi T, Komuro T. Age estimation using microfocus X-ray computed tomography of lower premolars. Forensic Science International. 2010;**200**:35-40. DOI: 10.1016/j.forsciint.2010.03.024

[88] Willems G. Dental age estimation and computers. In: Proceedings of the European IOFOS Millienium Meeting Leuven. Forensic Odontology; 23-26 August 2000; Leuven, Belgium. 2000. pp. 161–175

[89] Marroquina TY, Karkhanisa S, Kvaalb SI, Vasudavanc S, Krugera E, Tennant M. Age estimation in adults by dental imaging assessment systematic review. Forensic Science International. 2017;**275**:203-211. DOI: 10.1016/j.forsciint.2017.03.007

[90] Cameriere R, De Luca S, Egidi N, Bacaloni M, Maponi P, Ferrante L, Cingolani M. Automatic age estimation in adults by analysis of canine pulp/tooth ratio: Preliminary results. Journal of Forensic Radiology and Imaging. 2015;**3**:61-66

[91] De Angelis D, Gaudio D, Guercini N, Cipriani F, Gibelli D, Caputi S, et al. Age estimation from canine volumes. La Radiologia Medica. 2015;**120**(8):731-736

[92] Gustafson G. Age determination on teeth. Journal of the American Dental Association (1939). 1950;**41**:45-54

[93] Dalitz GD. Age determination of adult human remains by teeth examination. Journal of the Forensic Science Society. 1962;**3**:11-21. DOI: 10.1111/j.1834-7819.1962.tb02625.x

[94] Bang G, Ramm E. Determination of age in humans from root dentin transparency. Acta Odontologica Scandinavica. 1970;**28**:3-35

[95] Maples WR. An improved technique using dental histology for estimation of adult age. Journal of Forensic Sciences. 1978;**23**:764-770

[96] Solheim T, Vonen A. Dental age estimation, quality assurance and age estimation of asylum seekers in Norway. Forensic Science International. 2006;**159**:56-60. DOI: 10.1016/j.forsciint.2006.02.016

[97] Thoma KH. Oral Pathology. 2nd ed. St. Louis: CV Mosby Co; 1944

[98] Lamendin H. Age determination with the "simplified" Gustafson method. Le Chirurgien-Dentiste de France. 1988;**19**(58):43-47

[99] French VE, Baccino E, Sinfield L, Colomb S, Baum TP, Martrille L. Technical note: The two step procedure [TSP] for the determination of age at death of adult human remains in forensic cases. Forensic Science International. 2014;**244**:247-251. DOI: 10.1016/j.forsciint.2014.09.005

[100] Stack MV. A gravimetric study of crown growth rate of the human deciduous dentition. Biologia Neonatorum. 1964;**6**:197-224

[101] Deutsch D, Pe'er E, Gedalia I. Changes in size, morphology and weight of human anterior teeth during the fetal period. Growth. 1984;**48**:74-85

[102] Stavrionas C, Mastagas D, Stavrianou I, Karaiskou O. Dental age estimation of adults: A review of methods and principals. Research Journal of Medical Sciences. 2008;**2**:258-268. DOI: rjmsci.2008.258.268

[103] Kosa F, Antal A, Farkas I. Electron probe microanalysis of human teeth for the determination of individual age. Medicine, Science, and the Law. 1990;**30**:109-114

[104] Ohtani S, Ito R, Yamamoto T. Differences in the D/L aspartic acid ratios in dentin among different types of teeth from the same individual and estimated age. International Journal of Legal Medicine. 2003;**117**(3):149-152. DOI: 10.1007/s00414-003-0365-8

[105] Ogino T, Ogino H, Nagy B. Application of aspartic acid racemisation to forensic odontology: Post mortem designation of age at death. Forensic Science International. 1985;**29**:259-267

[106] Ritz-Timme S, Cattaneo C, Collins MJ, Waite ER, Schütz HW, Kaatsch HJ, Borrman HI. Age estimation: The state of the art in relation to the specific demands of forensic practice. International Journal of Legal Medicine. 2000;**113**:129-136

[107] Karkhanis S, Mack P, Franklin D. Age estimation standards for a Western Australian population using the dental age estimation technique developed by Kvaal et al. Forensic Science International. 2014;**235**:104.e1-104.e6. DOI: 10.1016/j.forsciint.2013.12.008

[108] Ohtani S, Hiroshi O, Asaka W. Estimation of age from teeth by amino acid racemisation influence of fixative. Journal of Forensic Sciences. 1997;**42**:137-139

[109] Helfman PM, Bada JL. Aspartic acid racemization in tooth enamel from living humans. Proceedings of the National Academy of Sciences of the United States of America. 1975;**72**:2891-2894

[110] Ritz S, Stock R, Schütz HW, Kaatsch HJ. Age estimation in biopsy specimens of dentin. International Journal of Legal Medicine. 1995;**108**:135-139

[111] Janardhanan M, Umadethan B, Biniraj KR, Kumar RB, Rakesh S. Neonatal line as a linear evidence of live birth: Estimation of postnatal survival of new born from primary tooth germs. Journal of Forensic Dental Sciences. 2011;**3**:8-13. DOI: 10.4103/0975-1475.85284

[112] Stavrianos C, Papadopoulos C, Vasiliadis L, Dagkalis P, Stavrianou I, Petalotis N. Enamel structure and forensic use. Research Journal of Biological Sciences. 2010;**5**:650-655. DOI: 10.3923/rjbsci.2010.650.655

[113] Birch W, Dean C. Rates of enamel formation in human deciduous dentition. Frontiers of Oral Biology. 2009;**13**:116-120. DOI: 10.1159/000242402

[114] Risnes S. Growth tracts in dental enamel. Journal of Human Evolution. 1998;**35**:331-350. DOI: 10.1006/jhev.1998.0229

[115] Naylor JW, Miller WG, Stokes GN, Stott GG. Cemental annulation enhancement: A technique for age determination in man. American Journal of Physical Anthropology. 1985;**68**:197-200. DOI: 10.1002/ajpa.1330680206

[116] Miller CS, Dove SB, Cottone JA. Failure of use of cemental annulations in teeth to determine the age of humans. Journal of Forensic Science. 1988;**33**:137-143

[117] Ge ZP, Ma RH, Li G, Zhang JZ, Ma XC. Age estimation based on pulp chamber volume of first molars from cone-beam computed tomography images. Forensic Science International. 2015 Aug;**253**:133.e1-133.e7. DOI: 10.1016/j.forsciint.2015.05.004

[118] Ge ZP, Yang P, Li G, Zhang JZ, Ma XC. Age estimation based on pulp cavity/chamber volume of 13 types of tooth from cone beam computed tomography images. International Journal of Legal Medicine. 2016 Jul;**130**(4):1159-1167. DOI: 10.1007/s00414-016-1384-6

[119] Baumrind S, Korn EL, Boyd RL. Apical root resorption in orthodontically treated adults. American Journal of Orthodontics and Dentofacial Orthopedics. 1996 Sep;**110**(3): 311-320

[120] Venkatesh S, Ajmera S, Ganeshkar SV. Volumetric pulp changes after orthodontic treatment determined by cone-beam computed tomography. Journal of Endodontia. 2014 Nov;**40**(11):1758-1763. DOI: 10.1016/j.joen.2014.07.029

[121] Marroquin Penaloza TY, Karkhanis S, Kvaal SI, Vasudavan S, Castelblanco E, Kruger E, Tennant M. Orthodontic treatment: Real risk for dental age estimation in adults? Journal of Forensic Sciences. 2017;**62**(4):907-910. DOI: 10.1111/1556-4029.13371

Chapter 7

Forensic DNA Technological Advancements as an Emerging Perspective on Medico-Legal Autopsy: A Mini Review

Zsolt Pádár, Petra Zenke and Zsolt Kozma

Additional information is available at the end of the chapter

http://dx.doi.org/10.5772/intechopen.72851

Abstract

The importance of biological traces and evidences related to a criminal matter has been recognized for a long time. The examination of the expression of genetic polymorphism has been an integral part of the multidisciplinary field of medico-legal autopsy for over a century. Since the initial application of blood group antigens for personalization of a putative perpetrator in a murder case, the discipline of forensic genetics has evolved as a standard of forensic sciences. The real breakthrough, the application of molecular tools and processes for the in-vitro replication of genetic substances, has increasingly allowed the exploitation of advances of molecular genetics for both forensic and criminal investigations. Although there are certainly many more applications and scientific fields in the medico-legal arena, the relatively fast progress of genetics, which has accelerated recently with state-of-art technologies, can provide ever more relevant information in relation to a corpse or the cause and manner that resulted in the corpse for autopsy. This topic concerns the currently accepted forensic DNA technology, and the last section reviews commonly used markers for nuclear and mitochondrial DNA analysis as well as ongoing research. This review also focuses on the increasingly important non-human sources of DNA, and shortly covers the main aspects of animal forensic DNA examination.

Keywords: forensic genetics, genetic identification, DNA typing, non-human DNA, animal forensics

1. Introduction

The application of genetics using molecular tools to characterize, identify or practically individualize the biological evidence after the medico-legal autopsy has been adopted worldwide [1].

Forensic genetics as an applied science provides those techniques to contribute to the proper examination of different collected samples. The range of associated biological evidence can be fairly wide, including samples from the body and on the body, as well as human and non-human biological remains. In spite of the existing sampling protocols or recommendations, in some situations, optimal sample collection may be pointless. In some cases, the swabbing of skin surface or fingernails can be effective [2–4] but also reveal an uninformative or uninterpretable mixture. In other cases, the optimal sampling tries to avoid an excessive number of samples, but the efficiency of seemly appropriate samples can vary according to subsequent analytical steps taken [5] or if the samples were provided for another type of examination [6, 7]. In essence, optimal solutions may be successfully obtained by using slightly different procedures depending on the source of the biological samples [8].

The methodology, in order to obtain genetic profiles, haplotypes, specific markers or species specific information, covers examination of both the nuclear and mitochondrial genome. The technical and theoretical foundation of forensic DNA analysis includes formal protocols as well as the use of standard, commercially available kits and reagents to obtain consensus examinations [9]. The desire for development of higher throughput of laboratory examination, the automation and standardization of steps of DNA analysis—the sample preparation/DNA extraction [10, 11], quantitation [12, 13], new devices [11, 14, 15] and yearly new multiplexes [9] for PCR amplification, fluorescent dye detection systems—provides for wide range advantages of its application.

However, despite the evolution in sensitivity and resolution of DNA techniques allowed by significant achievements year after year, the reality of cases present great risk and do have limitations. Although extreme applications and challenges such as low copy number [16, 17], degradation of DNA [18, 19] as well as mixtures [20, 21] or the collective consequences of these can present themselves as fairly complex issues, there is movement toward improving their interpretation [22, 23].

2. Brief insight into the past, present and future of forensic DNA technological advancements

Forensic genetic analysis is routinely used to obtain required information from biological samples of an autopsy for identification of persons associated with criminal casework or in instances of mass disaster. Upon the characterization of DNA samples using the most promising methods and techniques to improve their collection and further examinations via a medico-legal autopsy, the following steps of a DNA examination are performed in a molecular genetic laboratory, which is a significantly different environment from that of the autopsy room, for extraction, amplification, analyzing (profiling) and interpretation of samples. The proper process of sampling and sample storage used in an autopsy most certainly apply to the transportation of samples; however, contamination issues are always present, not only during the autopsy procedure, but also during the DNA analysis.

Several changes in methodology have promoted the genetic examination of samples with the desire to generate information from the smallest possible amounts of DNA. Wide-scale DNA extraction methods are commonly utilized in forensic practice, but have often proven to be insufficient in recovering all of the collected DNA. In many cases, however, this fact is irrelevant, due to the low minimal requirement of most common typing systems. Recently developed, commercially available kits and methodologies are optimized for specific types of samples and robotic systems [24, 25]. The adequate PCR-based methodologies [26–28] allowed for successful analysis from types of samples not previously examined, such as old, burnt, degraded bone and tissue samples [18, 29–31], single human hairs [32, 33], fingernail [2, 3, 34, 35], bite marks/saliva [36, 37] or touched surfaces [38, 39] and nonhuman remains [40].

2.1. DNA analysis of human and human-derived biological samples

2.1.1. Extraction of biological remains for DNA typing

As mentioned above, potential sources of biological samples related to autopsy are fairly wide ranging. The collected samples contain several substances in addition to DNA, therefore DNA molecules have to be separated from proteins and other cellular material as well as possible additional environmental contaminators, which can inhibit the subsequent steps of analysis [8].

For this reason, a number of methods have been steadily improved, upgrading the primary application for purification of DNA and avoiding its further degradation [10, 11]. Owing to the great variability of multiple influential factors, there can be no "best preparative answer," rather a selection of most suitable ones. A suitable extraction method should be consistent, sensitive and preferably quick and easy to use. It must also be able to deliver as-pure-as-possible DNA samples, ready to be used in downstream molecular applications and should pose minimum risk for possible cross-contamination between samples as well as between samples and users.

The solution-based, organic extraction method variants [41, 42], combined with filtration and concentration devices [43–45], have been used in practice for long time [46]. These methods can obtain high-quality DNA/RNA, and are adaptable for smaller or larger pieces of evidence material, but are relatively time consuming and require several—including some hazardous—chemicals and transfers. Higher-throughput automated DNA analysis promoted the benefits of variants of solid-phase DNA extraction methods [47]. The developed techniques include, for example, employing silica columns for the isolation and formation of complexes between nucleic acid and the silica gel matrix. In these the DNA selectively binds under particular pH and salt content conditions based on the principles of hydrogen binding to a hydrophilic matrix, ionic exchange using an anion exchanger or size exclusion and affinity. The retained DNA is finally eluted from other components in the subsequent washing steps [48]. An alternative, widely-used solid-phase DNA extraction method is based on an anion exchange/chelating resin that has a high affinity for polyvalent metal ions [41]. This procedure is less compound and faster and limits the use of multiple transfer tubes which reduces the risk of contamination. It requires only small sample volumes, and while it may be combined with, for example, proteinase K digestion and incubation, the high-temperature Chelex denatures the double-stranded DNA. Single-stranded DNA is obtained and remains suspended in the supernatant for downstream PCR [49–51]. Another commonly supplied solid-phase extraction is based on the reversible bonding of DNA to magnetic particles coated with a matrix of polymers or silica with terminal functionalized groups. The DNA bonded magnetic pellet is immobilized using an external magnet, and the discarded DNA are eluted after washing steps [52, 53]. Several commercially available extraction kits have been manufactured using the liquid/solid DNA extraction approach, and these have been incorporated into semi- and fully automated equipment [8, 24, 25, 54, 55]. The desired optimal DNA extraction from minute samples integrated with new technical developments and automation, "sample-in-answer" platforms for various types of tissues, are ongoing research topics [11, 14, 15, 56–58].

2.1.1.1. Extraction of compound and/or challenging samples

In point of fact, many—sometimes most—relevant casework samples belong to, so-called, difficult or challenging samples, which are, for example, more or less mixed and/or have a low copy number (LCN) or include low-template DNA (LTDNA). To process these difficult samples, several approaches have been developed, although the basic idea has not changed much. What would be the optimal selective or differential way of extraction in order to provide the greatest amount of the available target DNA with the least of the potential inhibitors and thus avoid downstream profiling from non-relevant allelic contributors [8]? An early technical solution for the separation of male and female content from mixed samples of sexual assault cases is based on the differential analyses of sperm and vaginal epithelial cells [59, 60]. The traditional differential extraction procedure has undergone modification, improvement and automated platforms, despite improvements in the alternative separation developments, and years later, is still in use today [61, 62].

Other potentially non-mixed, but easily containable low template DNA samples such as burned body or tissue which was subjected to a high temperature [46, 63–65], formalin-fixed samples [66–68], a piece of short hair with no root [69], or fingerprints of a touched surface and body parts [38, 39, 70–72] often require special consideration. Depending on the complexity of various influences, and with lack of valid information concerning the initial environmental circumstances and the chemical and/or physical processes involved, the degree of damage of and/or quality of obtained DNA cannot be, at first, accurately predicted. Since most extraction methods vary in relative efficiency and are incapable of offering an all-encompassing solution to the problem, for the purpose of optimization of a given procedure, it would be reasonable to consider the modification, combination or elimination of certain steps from different methodologies, specifically for trace samples [72].

2.1.2. DNA typing of human and human-derived biological samples of a medico-legal autopsy

2.1.2.1. Quantitation, amplification, sequencing, separation and detection

Although the practice of omitting the extraction and quantitation steps may occasionally seem to present a kind of benefit in regards to time and reduction of costs, for example in the case of disaster-victims [73], there may be multiple reasons for quantitation of the target DNA of extracted samples [13]. When it cannot be excluded that the extracted samples putatively include additional DNA from other species, or the seemly homogeneous sample is actually a mixed—for example, male and female epithelial cells at touched body surface—sample, determination of the appropriate amount of template DNA is required. In addition, the assumption that only low amounts of DNA obtainable in touched objects cannot always be correct, and in these situations, quantification can ensure the efficiency of downstream PCR [12]. It can help to provide an indication of hidden inhibitors [74] and to avoid off-scale artifacts or over-amplification. However, since the accuracy of various methods and commercially available kits can be slightly different [75–77], in cases of very low template amounts, quantitation can be often appropriated for indication, rather than merely an absolute measurement of the concentration, consequently, a negative quantitation result should not prevent future downstream amplification [12]. In light of standardized sampling tools and protocol developments as well as different alternative amplification methods—mainly in the field of reference samples—the importance of the quantitation step is partially based on ongoing research [78–80].

Very small amounts of nearly all targeted biological samples and DNA have been made detectable thanks to in-vitro replication—the polymerase chain reaction (PCR) [81]. The standardized amplification process, in increasing number of cycles, is an appropriate method to ensure efficient analysis, even of LTDNA obtained from the corpse belonging to persons other than that of the victim. The efficiency of PCR reaction is higher when the copy number of the entire target DNA is higher and/or the length of the amplified fragment is shorter. The specificity of PCR is directly affected by the primers and the primer binding site at target DNA. The number of markers can be amplified simultaneously in the same aliquot with an optimized mix of primer pairs, but the reaction can be inefficient due to the presence of different inhibitor molecules. When amplifying a low level of sample DNA—with higher probability of mixed samples—an unequal, stochastic fluctuation can manifest, which may lead to a preferential, imbalanced presence of the allelic component, and the number of PCR cycles cannot be increased unlimitedly [17, 82–84].

Since the initial application of the PCR method, several modifications and alternative molecules, e.g., novel DNA polymerases [85, 86], oligomeric mobility modifiers [87, 88] and fluorophores for labeling [89, 90], nonamers, aptamers [91, 92], etc., have been developed [82]. PCR can performed in a solution, using immobilized amplicon at solid phase (SP-PCR) [93, 94] or compartmentalization of template molecules in water droplets in a water-in-oil emulsion (Em-PCR) [92, 95, 96] to obtain the desired sequence or fragment length of sample DNA. The combination of improvements in chemistry and the evolution in analytical—separation, detection—platforms provides a plethora of applications. Merging advantages of fluorescent tags with mobility modifiers gives a unique electrophoretic signature for each amplified ligation product and enables extensive sample multiplexing for separation by capillary array electrophoresis with laser-induced fluorescence detection on an automated genetic analyzer [82, 97, 98]. The uses of fluorophores sensitized by fluorescence resonance energy transfer (FRET) provided detection kinetics of fluorescence accumulation, and combined PCR amplification with real-time detection [76, 77, 99, 100]. Alternative, or engineered, high-processivity DNA polymerases can have increased resistance to inhibitory factors relating to amplification of target DNA directly from samples without prior extraction or quantification [73, 78, 101, 102].

With the incorporation of more fluorophores as fluorescently labeled ddNTPs with primer extension and chain termination [103] on capillary electrophoresis platforms, a complete genome is sequenceable. An alternative solution for sequence determination is based on sequentially added nucleotides to the synthesis reaction, and real-time detection of an optical signal of released pyrophosphate molecules [104]. Recently, successive generations of massively parallel (MPS) or deep-sequencing methods—also referred to as next (NGS) or current generation sequencing—applying different phase PCR, different molecule-labeling, different—optical, proton or electric—signaling and platforms have revolutionized genomic research. State-of-the-art devices provide sequencing of both whole genomes and that of many individuals simultaneously, even from a single molecule of deoxyribonucleic acid [105–107]. As a result of variance in the error rate of existing MPS assays, platforms and computational techniques, forensic validation of the quality of a NGS provided data is recommended [106]. With the application of MPS technology in the forensic genetic field, the limited number of STR and SNP capable of being [108] can be ignored, while increasing the potent application of SNPs in degraded samples, allowing the simultaneous analysis of different marker types and improving the high throughput for mitochondrial DNA testing as well in caseworking and databasing for laboratories [109]. Additionally, the implementation of MPS on the field of molecular autopsy can increase the genomic and etiological background in cases of sudden death, allowing for new therapies and strategies for treatment or prevention [110]. Although new developments have mostly superseded conventional sequencing, the first-generation Sanger sequencing method is still occasionally used in many, not-only-lower throughput laboratories [111].

Over the last decade, microfluidic DNA analysis and devices—also referred as microfluidic biochips; sample-in to results-out, lab-on-a-chip (LOC) technology—present an enticing technology platform for automating laboratory procedures [112]. DNA biochips enable the miniaturization, integration, and automation of tests, and can perform thousands of biological reactions in a few seconds [113–115]. Integrated and mobile rapid-DNA devices, which are designed for several purposes, can produce quality STR-profiles suitable for reference or as database samples [80, 116]. The ever smaller size of state-of-the-art devices may allow for portable DNA analysis, possibly even meeting the needs of decentralized environments [79]. Despite successful typing results from casework samples which indicate that mobile technologies can provide investigative leads, their implementation in casework also brings along possible risks of losing information concerning crime scene sample profiling [117, 118]. Although the constantly increasing demand for high-throughput and parallel analytical devices assists integration of state-of-the-art technology with the forensic DNA process, many opportunities exist for further improvements.

2.1.2.2. Brief history of markers for individualization of human samples

Those genetic markers which have high mutation rates are appropriately polymorphic and useful for forensic examinations. Polymorphic DNA variation can be fundamentally divided into the branches of sequence polymorphic and length polymorphic markers or loci, both for human identity. The genome-scattered repeated DNA sequences form—sometimes referred as mini- or microsatellites [9, 119]—is typically designated by the length and number of repetitive units. The medium-length repeat (8–100 bp)—sometimes referred to as variable number of tandem repeat (VNTR)—markers such as D1S80, were mostly commonly used in the first part of the 1990s [120, 121]. Despite the relatively high level of polymorphisms of VNTR loci [122], the ability for easier PCR amplification—avoiding the problems of preferential amplification—has made the shorter-length repeat (2–6 bp)—sometimes referred to as microsatellites, short tandem repeat (STR)—markers more popular. The potency of analysis of degraded DNA using STR is greater due to it being less prone to allelic drop-out and more discriminative than the earlier alternatives.

A plethora of STRs are present in the human genome, and can vary not only in the length but also in the intervening sequence [123, 124]. Despite the complex, hypervariable motifs of some tetramer loci—posing a challenge for appropriate genotyping, among the types of STR markers—the tetranucleotide repetition has been developed for common forensic applications [9, 125–127]. Due to the narrow allele size range of STRs, the monoplex form of PCR has been rapidly replaced by the quadruplex form [9, 128–131]. The increasing number of standardized STR loci and fluorophore molecules combined with capillary electrophoretic separation [90, 97, 132, 133] has established the standard sets of STR markers for the forensic community [9]. Based on the national legislation of "core" loci, numerous national DNA databases have come into existence, and a collaboration on an international level between them has evolved. Existence of databases efficiently supports the recent state-of-the-art developments using database-related markers in further applications [9, 79, 80]. In addition to the application of MPS technology, it may also provide further sequence information for a more in-depth evaluation of STR alleles [106, 109, 134].

The early application of sequence polymorph markers in the forensic field is based on reverse dot-blot hybridization and allele-specific oligonucleotide (ASO) probes [135]. However, there are countries where the use of information of the coding DNA sequences for forensic purposes are restricted in some jurisdictions, which has limited the widespread use of sequence polymorphic markers in the forensic field. Additionally, the multi-allelic polymorphic STR markers have a higher number of possible alleles and a higher discrimination power than that of the early developed sequence polymorph systems such as Polymarker or HLA DQ alpha testing kits [136–138]. In spite of the validation and popularity of these types of polymorphic markers, they have already been phased out of forensic practice.

However, alternative sequence variability and biallelic markers—also referred to as single nucleotide substitution or polymorphisms (SNP)—are the most abundant polymorphism at the genome level, and they provide potent applications in forensic identification [139]. The biallelic polymorphisms have a lower mutation rate than the STRs [140, 141], and can be preferable in case of degraded samples. In spite of the lower discrimination power of a single biallelic marker when compared to a single STR locus, the increased number of simultaneously analyzed SNP loci can be effective for various uses in the forensic genetic field, which in light of advances in massive parallel sequencing can be especially progressive [109, 142–144].

2.1.2.3. Brief history of uniparental lineage markers

The Y-chromosome and mitochondrial DNA (mtDNA)—also referred as uniparental/lineage markers—are both haploid entities and, as such, are transmitted from generation to generation without recombination. Consequently, the variability of these markers depends on mutation events [145, 146]. The early implementation of these markers into forensic practice is based on several approaches and is becoming ubiquitous in forensic genetics [147, 148]. Although forensic application of these markers is accompanied by both advantages as well as limitations, their usage does, however, overcome two major challenges commonly encountered by the forensic scientist. In particular, for Y-chromosome specific markers, an increase in the otherwise-limited success of PCR obtained from male/female mixtures and, for mtDNA, obtaining genetic information from samples that are degraded, or nuclear DNA (nuDNA) free.

Although, in numerous cases, jurisdictions make use of the benefits that lineage marker analysis can bring, they do however have strong limitations in forensic applications, specifically, conclusions may not be drawn on the individual level as would be otherwise desirable [149–151]. Although haplotype markers usually are not included as standard markers in police databases, similarly to the Internet-based STR information resource [9, 152], haplotype databases have also been designed to store haplotypes from global populations. These provide a basis for frequency estimations and support data quality requirements to facilitate on-going efforts in forensics DNA investigation [153, 154]. In addition to complete autosomal genetic profiling, the genetic information of lineage markers is especially important in both forensic parental or kinship analyses [155], as well as from an evolutionary and genealogy point of view, in the prediction of potential geographic or ancestral origin [156–158].

The Y-chromosome [159], however, is present with only one copy per normal cell, and has higher diversity than mtDNA in addition to an increasing number of Y-STRs [9, 155, 160] completed by rapidly mutating (RM) markers [155, 160–162], Y-SNPs [155, 160, 163–165] and insertion/deletion polymorph (Indel) markers [166, 167]. Although, the analysis of Y-chromosomal markers can provide complementary information in addition to an autosomal genetic profile [168], the most common application of Y-STRs is in cases of sexual assault, when the female component can greatly overshadow the male component, making autosomal STR profiling frequently difficult, unclear or impossible. Examination of Y-chromosome markers is available in a wide range of commercial kits [12, 169, 170] which perform adequately for identifying male lineages.

Mitochondrial DNA, similar to the Y-chromosome, is not a unique identifier, but its examination in criminal cases can be nevertheless reasonable, for example, when the profiling of nuclear DNA markers fails to produce a profile. The mitochondrial genome evolves relatively rapidly, and newly arising—primarily point—mutations tend to become fixed faster and at a higher rate than that for nuDNA. In the mitochondrial genome, the highest level of genetic variation is located in the control region (CR) [171]. The most common type of polymorphs belong to SNP, which can be found not only in the hypervariable regions (HV I–III), but in the entire mtDNA genome as well [172, 173]. Single base mutations may lead to such a condition in which both the mutated and original forms coexist as admixture, which is referred to as heteroplasmy [174–176]. Similarly, indel variability is also present in the mitochondrial genome [177, 178]. The higher sensitivity resulting from the order of magnitudes copy number of mtDNA, compared to that of nuDNA, makes it possible to obtain reliable haplotypes, when the DNA gathered from samples is highly fragmented and/or damaged. In addition, due to the inheritance of molecules, the genetic information from maternal relatives as references, e.g., for an unknown or missing person, are suitable for making direct comparisons. In the field of forensic genetics, the mtDNA is also a so-called historical marker analyzed by Sanger sequencing technologies [179]. This method combined with capillary array instrumentation or the application of pyrosequencing technology was previously ubiquitous in laboratories [180, 181] and is currently still in use [182–184].

Although the highest-polymorph regions are the traditionally-analyzed hypervariable regions (HV I–III), in some cases, sequencing of the whole mitochondrial genome is capable of solving even those cases, in which the hypervariable haplotype cannot be differentiated between individuals. The increasing demand for mtDNA examination—missing person cases, natural disasters, human rights investigations, etc.—has revealed the limitation of throughput and cost-benefit relations of conventional technology which had previously focused on only part of the entire mitochondrial genome. The implementation of novel technologies such as MPS, provides an automated workflow and could offer its usage for a wide range of samples. Over the last decade, developments related to the sequencing of entire mtDNA genomes [185, 186] have resulted not only in the high throughput of data, improving the recovery of genetic information from forensic specimens, but have also focused on the discrimination potential of mtDNA evidence. Comparison of whole mitochondrial genomes can provide an understanding of mtDNA mutation and heteroplasmy, and completing it with the forensic validation of MPS platforms may lead to the deconvolution of mixtures, as well as providing solutions to other challenging casework problems [106, 187, 188].

2.1.2.4. Markers for investigation of cause or manner of death: molecular autopsy

Even though the active field of medico-legal autopsy can vary among different countries according to traditional and legislatorial backgrounds, the use of molecular analyses is becoming steadily more frequent and its importance is becoming more recognized in postmortem examinations. Several different forensic sciences—including forensic genetics—are inherently involved in this multidisciplinary molecular investigation. Molecular autopsy is still a relatively new concept in pathology and forensic sciences [189]. In contrast to cases of intentional or suspected violent death, in instances when death occurred either suddenly, unexpectedly, or involving infants and the young [3], autopsy sampling focuses on the corpse's own substances to aid in determination of genetic markers and mutations which could be responsible for the cause or manner of death. From this point of view, the use of forensic genetics is not only strictly limited to purposes of identification, but may also be tasked by performing genetic tests for genes associated with disease [190, 191].

Several specific or rare diseases may be linked to a particular pathological condition in cases of both positive and negative autopsy [189, 192]. Novel MPS technology can be highly informative in detection of all variants of genes affecting unexpected death in epilepsy, adverse drug reactions and metabolism [192–194], as well as the cardiovascular system, e.g., cardiomyopathies and cardiac ion channelopathies, which have been associated with sudden cardiac death [110, 195].

Molecular autopsy is an emerging part of the medico-legal autopsy, and with the incorporation of genome-wide data and computational techniques, its benefit to this multidisciplinary field should continue to increase [192].

2.1.2.5. Markers for supplemental information

An earlier phase in forensic examinations focused on polymorph markers for the construction of forensic databases, as they do not vary over time [196]. The numbers of STR marker-based, legislated databases and their cooperation at the transnational level, as well as the volume of associative data-records and their efficiency are considerable economic factors for their consolidation in forensic practice [197, 198]. Massive parallel sequencing (MPS) techniques have recently provided the opportunity to extend the contemporary investigative role of databases by the sequencing of STRs [199]. A plethora of markers have been recently introduced for forensic applications, although the majority of them have yet to be integrated into forensic databases. The level of polymorphisms is based upon new mutations, which, when they arise in a population, are spread via natural selection, migration and genetic drift. Different types of markers exhibit different rates of mutation; for example, indel mutations occur less frequently than single nucleotide substitutions in both nuclear and mitochondrial genomes [119, 134, 140, 141, 145, 159, 177, 178]. A large number of autosomal and sex-chromosomal STRs, SNPs from both nuclear and mitochondrial genomes, indels and ancestry-informative markers (AIMs) and mRNA and phenotypical markers (FDP) have been introduced and applied by the forensic community. Numerous new markers are being implemented in advancing the desired goals of investigative authorities, specifically, how forensic genetics can help to improve the collection of the most relevant information in terms of individualization and identification from the least amount of biological samples. Due to their abundant distribution in both the nuclear and mitochondrial genome, SNPs increasingly can provide the genetic background for the prediction of physical characteristics [200, 201], or geographical origin [202, 203], and can also provide investigative tools to trace unknown individuals [204, 205] even from historical remains [206–208]. Determination of ancestry [209, 210] and externally visible characteristics, such as skin, eye and hair pigmentation [211, 212], morphology [213, 214], or age [215, 216], is an ongoing research field of forensics, requiring both forensic validation of analytical platforms and computation data.

Although there is a distinct probability of encountering the artificially altered appearance of phenotypes, the phrase "DNA witness" has obtained new perspectives with its potential for providing information of higher accuracy than that of traditional eye witnesses. In light of the above, forensic DNA phenotyping (FDP), although a promising technique, raises multiple, not only scientific, but also ethical and legislative issues [217, 218].

2.2. DNA analysis of nonhuman remains

There are cases when the victims have been involved in a pet or livestock animal attack with fatal—usually unwitnessed—consequences [40, 219, 220]. In other cases, animal hair from a victim's body helps to reveal the perpetrator [221], or so-called "silent witnesses" such as plant remains [222] on corpses, or even evidence of algae from postmortem tissues, aid in determination of the manner of death [223]. Due to the increasingly particular importance of genetic analysis of nonhuman substances in these types of cases, forensic genetics today is progressively incorporating the examination of nonhuman genetic material to an ever greater extent [224]. In essence, the similarities in analog and ortholog variable components of genomes provide forensic investigation of nonhuman biological substances in the same manner as for human forensics, but distinctions existing in different organisms and species, i.e., genomic architectures, reproductive strategies and genetic diversity, are continuously broadening the dependent scientific areas. The benefits stemming from the extension of forensic genetics toward nonhuman relations were clearly recognized decades ago [225], and the incorporated application of animal, plant or microorganisms has been actualized in a large scale of caseworks, from animal attacks [226, 227] to bioterrorism [228], as well as in wildlife crimes [229, 230], identification of food composition [231, 232], *Cannabis sp.* chemotyping [233, 234], and even the estimation of postmortem interval and skin microbiomes [235, 236]. Other various aspects of possible nonhuman biological evidences found on the corpse, e.g., pollens or plant fragments, can reveal potential indirect links to the perpetrator, and also additional, case-related facts, complementing autopsy information with the modality of death or the crime scene setting for purposes of case reconstruction [237, 238]. The human-related techniques of forensic genetics have been adapted to nonhuman analyses, but the genetic markers implemented frequently originate from the field of conservation biology. This could be a reason that markers and data computation are more varied in nonhuman areas than those in human identification, and comparatively, are rarely standardized for all species. In recent years, genome-wide analyses and MPS technology have revolutionized this broad field in any case, so it would not be practical to introduce the enormous variety of nonhuman forensic DNA analysis here, within this section. Due to the common coexistence of humans and domestic animals, dog violence on humans leading to fatal consequences represents a frequent type of case [224, 239–242]. In these cases, DNA can be separated from saliva from within the biting area, from animal hairs and sometimes blood, or bitten material, including the victims' clothing [40, 219]. The saliva of dogs is a suitable source for DNA extraction [243–245], even when the human victim's blood is present [40, 219]. Although DNA extraction from dog hairs has similarly been solved using well-developed methods [246–249], genetic typing of single dog hairs has often failed [247]. As an analysis concept using shortened amplicons [231, 250, 251], the isolated DNA may be sufficient for successful amplification. Otherwise, when the amplification of nuclear markers is insufficient due to the low quantity and degradation of nuclear DNA, mitochondrial DNA may be more appropriate [252, 253].

STR-based genetic markers in multiplex forms have been continuously developed for canine individualization [254–257]. Due to the fact that dogs have been involved from relatively early on in the forensic genetic field, positive differences have been made for canines compared to other species in forensic applications. The quality requirement for implementation of canine DNA analysis in forensic practice is as ambitious as in human forensics. The STR marker-sets which have been developed have relevant population studies, occasionally extended with genetic variance [258–264], inbreeding [258, 261] and mutation data [265]. Sequence databases of canine mitochondrial DNA have also been developed [266–268].

Accreditation measures for DNA typing in the nonhuman or animal forensic [269] field are established on a different level, and are occasionally of significant importance, as the potential number of species could be incorporated into legal procedures in a myriad of ways. Although, primarily due to the inherent heterogeneity of existing laboratory environments and the expense and complexity of accreditation, equalization of the nonhuman field to human forensic genetics poses a monumental challenge. Nonetheless, the first steps toward this goal must obviously be taken according to the developed recommendations concerning the standardization of DNA typing of animal species and products [270–272].

3. Conclusions

Although considerably younger, the field of forensic genetics is a distinct part of the forensic arena [1] and its presence has become widespread and is now accepted as the primary forensic method for identifying persons of interest [273]. The modern implementation of genetic analysis within the wider-scale field of autopsy has brought with it an increase in the potentiality of exhibits. The accreditation and quality assurance of the field of forensic genetics, in accordance with professional recommendations [274], legal regulations and harmonization [275], quality standardization and systems [276], as well as the establishment of national and international databases and their subsequent cooperation [197], have caused genetics to occasionally play a pioneer role among scientific fields on the forensic palette. Despite the relative youth of forensic genetics, several generations of methods have already been developed and obsoleted in this field. Recently, sequencing techniques have continued to move ahead at a staggering speed, and the massive parallel sequencing strategy, capable of simultaneously generating thousands of reads on state-of-art devices, will revolutionize genetic analysis [277, 278]. Although the admissibility of MPS results in a court of law will most likely continue to be challenged—as are mostly newly introduced methods—foreseeably raising concerns about privacy [278], the complementary application of MPS genome-wide data, with other innovative and advanced analytical systems—e.g., imaging analysis—can extend the professionalism and efficiency of the multidisciplinary medico-legal field to the ultimate benefit of society [278].

Author details

Zsolt Pádár[1,2]*, Petra Zenke[3] and Zsolt Kozma[1]

*Address all correspondence to: drpadarzsolt@gmail.com

1 Department of Forensic Medicine, Medical School, University of Pécs, Hungary

2 Criminology and Forensic Research Centre, Széchenyi István University, Győr, Hungary

3 Department of Animal Breeding and Genetics, University of Veterinary Medicine, Budapest, Hungary

References

[1] Lynch M. God's signature: DNA profiling, the new gold standard in forensic science. Endeavour. 2003;**27**(2):93-97. DOI: 10.1016/S0160-9327(03)00068-1

[2] Wiegand P, Bajanowski T, Brinkmann B. DNA typing of debris from fingernails. International Journal of Legal Medicine. 1993;**106**:81-83. DOI: 10.1007/BF01225045

[3] Padar Z, Barta A, Egyed B. et al. Hungarian experience of examination of the fingernails in violent crime. In: Sensabaugh GF, Lincoln P, Olaisen B, editors. Progress in Forensic Genetics 8: Proceedings of the 18th International ISFH Congress; 17–21 August 1999; San Francisco, CA, USA. Amsterdam, Lausanne, New York: Elsevier (ICS 1193); 2000. pp. 492-494. ISBN: 978-0444503039

[4] Flanagan N, McAlister C. The transfer and persistence of DNA under the fingernails following digital penetration of the vagina. Forensic Science International. Genetics. 2011;**5**(5):479-483. DOI: 10.1016/j.fsigen.2010.10.008

[5] Hoff-Olsen P, Mevag B, Staalstrøm E, et al. Extraction of DNA from decomposed human tissue. An evaluation of five extraction methods for short tandem repeat typing. Forensic Science International. 1999;**105**(3):171-183. DOI: https://doi.org/10.1016/S0379-0738(99)00128-0

[6] Reshef A, Barash M, Voskoboinik L, et al. STR typing of formalin-fixed paraffin embedded (FFPE) aborted foetal tissue in criminal paternity cases. Science & Justice. 2011;**51**(1):19-23. DOI: 10.1016/j.scijus.2010.09.001

[7] Patel PG, Selvarajah S, Boursalie S, et al. Preparation of formalin-fixed paraffin-embedded tissue cores for both RNA and DNA extraction. Journal of Visualized Experiments. 2016;**114**:54299. DOI: 10.3791/54299

[8] Butler JM. Chapter 2—DNA Extraction Methods. In: Advanced Topics in Forensic DNA Typing: Methodology. Waltham, San Diego: Academic Press; 2012. pp. 29-47. ISBN: 978-0-12-374513-2. DOI: 10.1016/B978-0-12-374513-2.00002-6

[9] The National Institute of Justice. Standard Reference Database SRD 130, Short Tandem Repeat DNA Internet DataBase. [Internet]. Available from: http://strbase.nist.gov [Accessed: 2017.10.10]

[10] Stray JE, Liu JY, Brevnov MG, Shewale JG. Extraction of DNA from forensic biological samples for genotyping. In: Stray JE, editor. Forensic DNA Analysis. Current Practices and Emerging Technologies. Boca Raton, London, New York: CRC Press; 2013. pp. 39-64. ISBN: 978-1-4665-7136-5. DOI: 10.1201/b15361-5

[11] Gan W, Zhuang B, Zhang P, et al. A filter paper-based microdevice for low-cost, rapid, and automated DNA extraction and amplification from diverse sample types. Lab on a Chip. 2014;**14**(19):3719-3728. DOI: 10.1039/c4lc00686k

[12] Van Oorschot RAH, Ballantyne KN, Mitchell RJ. Forensic trace DNA: A review. Investigative Genetics. 2010;**1**:14. DOI: 10.1186/2041-2223-1-14

[13] Lee SB, McCord B, Buel E. Advances in forensic DNA quantification: A review. Electrophoresis. 2014;**35**(21–22):3044-3052. DOI: 10.1002/elps.201400187

[14] Lounsbury JA, Karlsson A, Miranian DC, et al. From sample to PCR product in under 45 minutes: A polymeric integrated microdevice for clinical and forensic DNA analysis. Lab on a Chip. 2013;**13**(7):1384-1393. DOI: 10.1039/c3lc41326h

[15] Cox JO, DeCarmen TS, Ouyang Y, et al. A novel, integrated forensic microdevice on a rotation-driven platform: Buccal swab to STR product in less than 2 h. Electrophoresis. 2016;**37**(23–24):3046-3058. DOI: 10.1002/elps.201600307

[16] Budowle B, Eisenberg AJ, van Daal A. Validity of low copy number typing and applications to forensic science. Croatian Medical Journal. 2009;**50**(3):207-217. DOI: 10.3325/cmj.2009.50.207

[17] Butler JM. Chapter 11—Low-level DNA testing: Issues, concerns, and solutions. In: Advanced Topics in Forensic DNA Typing: Methodology. Waltham, San Diego: Academic Press; 2012. pp. 311-346. ISBN: 978-0-12-374513-2. DOI: 10.1016/B978-0-12-374513-2.00011-7

[18] Alaeddini R, Walsh SJ, Abbas A. Forensic implications of genetic analyses from degraded DNA—A review. Forensic Science International. Genetics. 2010;**4**(3):148-157. DOI: 10.1016/j.fsigen.2009.09.007

[19] Tvedebrink T, Eriksen PS, Mogensen HS, Morling N. Statistical model for degraded DNA samples and adjusted probabilities for allelic drop-out. Forensic Science International. Genetics. 2012;**6**(1):97-101. DOI: 10.1016/j.fsigen.2011.03.001

[20] Gill P, Brenner CH, Buckleton JS, et al. DNA commission of the International Society of Forensic Genetics: Recommendations on the interpretation of mixtures. Forensic Science International. 2006;**160**(2–3):90-101. DOI: 10.1016/j.forsciint.2006.04.009

[21] Tvedebrink T, Eriksen PS, Mogensen HS, Morling N. Identifying contributors of DNA mixtures by means of quantitative information of STR typing. Journal of Computational Biology. 2012;**19**(7):887-902. DOI: 10.1089/cmb.2010.0055

[22] Gill P, Gusmão L, Haned H, Mayr WR, et al. DNA commission of the International Society of Forensic Genetics: Recommendations on the evaluation of STR typing results that may include drop-out and/or drop-in using probabilistic methods. Forensic Science International. Genetics. 2012;**6**(6):679-688. DOI: 10.1016/j.fsigen.2012.06.002

[23] Pascali V, Prinz M. Highlights of the conference 'The hidden side of DNA profiles: Artifacts, errors and uncertain evidence'. Forensic Science International. Genetics. 2012; **6**(6):775-777. DOI: 10.1016/j.fsigen.2012.08.011

[24] Greenspoon SA, Ban JD, Sykes K, et al. Application of the BioMek 2000 Laboratory Automation Workstation and the DNA IQ System to the extraction of forensic casework samples. Journal of Forensic Sciences. 2004;**49**:29-39. DOI: 10.1520/JFS2003179

[25] Frégeau CJ, Lett CM, Fourney RM. Validation of a DNA IQ™-based extraction method for TECAN robotic liquid handling workstations for processing casework. Forensic Science International. Genetics. 2010;**4**:292-304. DOI: 10.1016/j.fsigen.2009.11.001

[26] Wiegand P, Kleiber M. Less is more—Length reduction of STR amplicons using redesigned primers. International Journal of Legal Medicine. 2001;**114**:285-287. DOI: 10.1007/s004140000162

[27] Grubwieser P, Mühlmann R, Berger B, et al. A new "mini-STR-multiplex" displaying reduced amplicon lengths for the analysis of degraded DNA. International Journal of Legal Medicine. 2006;**120**:115-120. DOI: 10.1007/s00414-005-0013-6

[28] Parsons TJ, Huel R, Davoren J, et al. Application of novel 'mini-amplicon' STR multiplexes to high volume casework on degraded skeletal remains. Forensic Science International. Genetics. 2007;**1**:175-179. DOI: 10.1016/j.fsigen.2007.02.003

[29] Primorac D, Andelinovic S, Definis-Gojanovic M, et al. Identification of war victims from mass graves in Croatia, Bosnia and Herzegovina by the use of standard forensic methods and DNA testing. Journal of Forensic Sciences. 1996;**41**:891-894. DOI: 10.1520/JFS14019J

[30] Baeta M, Núñez C, Cardoso S, et al. Digging up the recent Spanish memory: Genetic identification of human remains from mass graves of the Spanish Civil War and posterior dictatorship. Forensic Science International. Genetics. 2015;**19**:272-279. DOI: 10.1016/j.fsigen.2015.09.001

[31] Ossowski A, Diepenbroek M, Zwolski M, et al. A case study of an unknown mass grave —Hostages killed 70 years ago by a Nazi firing squad identified thanks to genetics. Forensic Science International. 2017;**278**:173-176. DOI: 10.1016/j.forsciint.2017.06.038

[32] Hellman A, Rohleder U, Schmitter H, Wittig M. STR typing of human telogen hairs—A new approach. International Journal of Legal Medicine. 2001;**114**:269-273. DOI: 10.1007/s004140000175

[33] Grzybowski T, Malyarchuk B, Czarny J, et al. High levels of mitochondrial DNA heteroplasmy in single hair roots: Reanalysis and revision. Electrophoresis. 2003;**24**(7–8): 1159-1165. DOI: 10.1002/elps.200390149

[34] Matte M, Williams L, Frappier R, Newman J. Prevalence and persistence of foreign DNA beneath fingernails. Forensic Science International. Genetics. 2012;**6**(2):236-243. DOI: 10.1016/j.fsigen.2011.05.008

[35] Ottens R, Taylor D, Linacre A. DNA profiles from fingernails using direct PCR. Forensic Science, Medicine, and Pathology. 2015;**11**:99. DOI: 10.1007/s12024-014-9626-8

[36] Sweet D, Lorente JA, Valenzuela A, et al. PCR-based DNA typing of saliva stains recovered from human skin. Journal of Forensic Sciences. 1997;**42**:447-451. DOI: 10.1520/JFS14146J

[37] Kenna J, Smyth M, McKenna L, et al. The recovery and persistence of salivary DNA on human skin. Journal of Forensic Sciences. 2011;**56**(1):170-175. DOI: 10.1111/j.1556-4029.2010.01520.x

[38] Van Oorschot RAH, Jones MK. DNA fingerprints from fingerprints. Nature. 1997;**387**: 767. DOI: 10.1038/42838

[39] Wiegand P, Kleiber M. DNA typing of epithelial cells after strangulation. International Journal of Legal Medicine. 1997;**110**(4):181-183. DOI: 10.1007/s004140050063

[40] Eichmann C, Berger B, Reinhold M, et al. Canine-specific STR typing of saliva traces on dog bite wounds. International Journal of Legal Medicine. 2004;**118**:337-342. DOI: 10.1007/s00414-004-0479-7

[41] Sambrook J, Fritsch EF, Maniatis T. Molecular Cloning: A Laboratory Manual. New York: CSHL Press; 1989. ISBN 0879693096

[42] Chomczynski P, Sacchi N. The single-step method of RNA isolation by acid guanidinium thiocyanate-phenol-chloroform extraction: Twenty-something years on. Nature Protocols. 2006;**1**(2):581-585. DOI: 10.1038/nprot.2006.83

[43] Comey C, Koons B, Presley K, et al. DNA extraction strategies for amplified fragment length polymorphism analysis. Journal of Forensic Sciences. 1994;**39**(5):1254-1269. DOI: 10.1520/JFS13711J

[44] Hudlow WR, Krieger R, Meusel M, et al. The NucleoSpin® DNA clean-up XS kit for the concentration and purification of genomic DNA extracts: An alternative to microdialysis filtration. Forensic Science International. Genetics. 2011;**5**(3):226-230. DOI: 10.1016/j.fsigen.2010.03.005

[45] Doran AE, Foran DR. Assessment and mitigation of DNA loss utilizing centrifugal filtration devices. Forensic Science International. Genetics. 2014;**13**:187-190. DOI: 10.1016/j.fsigen.2014.08.001

[46] Maciejewska A, Wlodarczyk R, Pawlowski R. The influence of high temperature on the possibility of DNA typing in various human tissues. Folia Histochemica et Cytobiologica. 2015;**53**(4):322-332. DOI: 10.5603/fhc.a2015.0029

[47] McCormick RM. A solid-phase extraction procedure for DNA purification. Analytical Biochemistry. 1989;**181**(1):66-74. DOI: 10.1016/0003-2697(89)90394-1

[48] Greenspoon SA, Scarpetta MA, Drayton ML, Turek SA. QIAamp spin columns as a method of DNA isolation for forensic casework. Journal of Forensic Sciences. 1998; **43**(5):1024-1030. DOI: 10.1520/JFS14351J

[49] Willard JM, Lee DA, Holland MM. Recovery of DNA for PCR amplification from blood and forensic samples using a chelating resin. Methods in Molecular Biology. 1998;**98**:9-18. DOI: 10.1385/0-89603-443-7:9

[50] Idris B, Goodwin W. Comparison of Chelex®-100 with two solid phase DNA extraction techniques. Forensic Science International: Genetics Supplement Series. 2015;**5**:e274-e275. DOI: 10.1016/j.fsigss.2015.09.109

[51] Pîrlea S, Puiu M, Răducan A, Oancea D. Permanganate-assisted removal of PCR inhibitors during the DNA Chelex extraction from stained denim samples. International Journal of Legal Medicine. 2017;**131**:323-331. DOI: 10.1007/s00414-016-1443-z

[52] Deggerdal A, Larsen F. Rapid isolation of PCR-ready DNA from blood, bone marrow and cultured cells, based on paramagnetic beads. BioTechniques. 1997 Mar;**22**(3):554-557

[53] Saiyed ZM, Bochiwal C, Gorasia H, et al. Application of magnetic particles (Fe_3O_4) for isolation of genomic DNA from mammalian cells. Analytical Biochemistry. 2006;**356**(2): 306-308. DOI: 10.1016/j.ab.2006.06.027

[54] Xenophontos S, Christofi V, Iosif G, et al. Internal validation of the QIAamp DNA Investigator Kit, QIAamp 96 DNA Swab BioRobot Kit and the BioRobot Universal System for DNA extraction from reference and crime scene samples. Forensic Science International. Genetics. 2015;**14**:e8-10. DOI: 10.1016/j.fsigen.2014.10.020

[55] Ip SC, Lin SW, Lai KM. An evaluation of the performance of five extraction methods: Chelex® 100, QIAamp® DNA Blood Mini Kit, QIAamp® DNA Investigator Kit, QIAsymphony® DNA Investigator® Kit and DNA IQ™. Science & Justice. 2015;**55**(3): 200-208. DOI: 10.1016/j.scijus.2015.01.005

[56] Le Roux D, Root BE, Hickey JA, et al. An integrated sample-in-answer-out microfluidic chip for rapid human identification by STR analysis, Lab on a Chip. 2014;**14**(22):4415-4425. DOI: 10.1039/c4lc00685b

[57] Shin Y, Swee YL, Lee TY, Park MK. Dimethyl adipimidate/thin film sample processing (DTS); a simple, low-cost, and versatile nucleic acid extraction assay for downstream analysis. Scientific Reports. 2015;**5**:4127. DOI: 10.1038/srep14127

[58] Gan W, Gu Y, Han J, Li CX. Chitosan-modified filter paper for nucleic acid extraction and "in situ PCR" on a thermoplastic microchip. Analytical Chemistry. 2017;**89**(6):3568-3575. DOI: 10.1021/acs.analchem.6b04882

[59] Wiegand P, Schürenkamp M, Schütte U. DNA extraction from mixtures of body fluid using mild preferential lysis. International Journal of Legal Medicine. 1992;**104**(6):359-360. DOI: 10.1007/BF01369558

[60] Yoshida K, Sekiguchi K, Mizuno N, et al. The modified method of two-step differential extraction of sperm and vaginal epithelial cell DNA from vaginal fluid mixed with semen. Forensic Science International. 1995;**72**(1):25-33. DOI: 10.1016/0379-0738(94)01668-U

[61] Lounsbury JA, Nambiar SM, Karlsson A, et al. Enhanced recovery of spermatozoa and comprehensive lysis of epithelial cells from sexual assault samples having a low cell counts or aged up to one year. Forensic Science International. Genetics. 2014;**8**(1):84-89. DOI: 10.1016/j.fsigen.2013.06.015

[62] Klein SB, Buoncristiani MR. Evaluating the efficacy of DNA differential extraction methods for sexual assault evidence. Forensic Science International. Genetics. 2017;**29**:109-117. DOI: 10.1016/j.fsigen.2017.03.021

[63] Caputo M, Irisarri M, Alechine E, Corach D. A DNA extraction method of small quantities of bone for high-quality genotyping. Forensic Science International. Genetics. 2013;**7**(5):488-493. DOI: 10.1016/j.fsigen.2013.05.002

[64] Damgaard PDB, Margaryan A, Schroeder H, et al. Improving access to endogenous DNA in ancient bones and teeth. Scientific Reports. 2015;**5**:11184. DOI: 10.1038/srep11184

[65] Uzair A, Rasool N, Wasim M. Evaluation of different methods for DNA extraction from human burnt bones and the generation of genetic profiles for identification. Medicine, Science, and the Law. 2017;**1**:25802417723808. DOI: 10.1177/0025802417723808

[66] Gilbert MT, Haselkorn T, Bunce M, et al. The isolation of nucleic acids from fixed, paraffin-embedded tissues-which methods are useful when? PLoS One. 2007;**20**(6):e537. DOI: 10.1371/journal.pone.0000537

[67] Tomonari K, Sonoda A, Ikehara A, et al. Comparison of methods for the extraction of DNA from formalin-fixed paraffin-embedded tissues for human identification. Japanese Journal of Forensic Science and Technology. 2017. Article ID: 734. DOI: http://doi.org/10.3408/jafst.734

[68] Reid KM, Maistry S, Ramesar R, Heathfield LJ. A review of the optimisation of the use of formalin fixed paraffin embedded tissue for molecular analysis in a forensic post-mortem setting. Forensic Science International. 2017;**280**:181-187. DOI: https://doi.org/10.1016/j.forsciint.2017.09.020

[69] Harper KA, Meiklejohn KA, Merritt RT, et al. Isolation of mitochondrial DNA from single, short hairs without roots using pressure cycling technology. SLAS Technology. 2018;**23**(1):97-105. DOI: 10.1177/2472630317732073

[70] Hebda LM, Doran AE, Foran DR. Collecting and analyzing DNA evidence from fingernails: A comparative study. Journal of Forensic Sciences. 2014;**59**(5):1343-1350. DOI: 10.1111/1556-4029.12465

[71] Ostojic L, Wurmbach E. Analysis of fingerprint samples, testing various conditions, for forensic DNA identification. Science & Justice. 2017;**57**(1):35-40. DOI: 10.1016/j.scijus.2016.08.009

[72] Solomon AD, Hytinen ME, McClain AM, et al. An optimized DNA analysis workflow for the sampling, extraction, and concentration of DNA obtained from archived latent fingerprints. Journal of Forensic Sciences. 2018;**63**(1):47-57. DOI: 10.1111/1556-4029.13504

[73] Habib M, Pierre-Noel A, Fogt F, et al. Direct amplification of biological evidence and DVI samples using the Qiagen investigator 24plex GO! Kit. Genetics. Forensic Science International: Genetics Supplement Series. 2017;**6**:e208-e210. DOI: 10.1016/j.fsigss.2017.09.079

[74] Moreno LI, McCord BR. The use of direct analysis in real time (DART) to assess the levels of inhibitors co-extracted with DNA and the associated impact in quantification and amplification. Electrophoresis. 2016;**37**(21):2807-2816. DOI: 10.1002/elps.201500480

[75] Kumar D, Panigrahi MK, Suryavanshi M, et al. Quantification of DNA extracted from formalin fixed paraffin-embeded tissue comparison of three techniques: Effect on PCR efficiency. Journal of Clinical and Diagnostic Research. 2016;**10**(9):BC01-BC03. DOI: 10.7860/JCDR/2016/19383.8407

[76] Goecker ZC, Swiontek SE, Lakhtakia A, Roy R. Comparison of Quantifiler(®) trio and InnoQuant™ human DNA quantification kits for detection of DNA degradation in developed and aged fingerprints. Forensic Science International. 2016;**263**:132-138. DOI: 10.1016/j.forsciint.2016.04.009

[77] Josefiova J, Matura R, Votrubova J, et al. Comparison of fluorometric and real-time PCR quantification of DNA extracted from formalin fixed tissue Forensic Science International: Genetics Supplement Series. 2017;**6**:e137-e139. DOI: http://dx.doi.org/10.1016/j.fsigss.2017.09.028

[78] Ambers A, Wiley R, Novroski N, Budowle B. Direct PCR amplification of DNA from human bloodstains, saliva, and touch samples collected with microFLOQ®swabs. Forensic Science International. Genetics. 2018;**32**:80-87. DOI: https://doi.org/10.1016/j.fsigen.2017.10.010

[79] Salceda S, Barican A, Buscaino J, et al. Validation of a rapid DNA process with the RapidHIT® ID system using GlobalFiler® express chemistry, a platform optimized for decentralized testing environments. Forensic Science International. Genetics. 2017;**28**:21-34. DOI: 10.1016/j.fsigen.2017.01.005

[80] Moreno LI, Brown AL, Callaghan TF. Internal validation of the DNAscan/ANDE™ rapid DNA analysis™ platform and its associated PowerPlex® 16 high content DNA biochip cassette for use as an expert system with reference buccal swabs. Forensic Science International. Genetics. 2017;**29**:100-108. DOI: 10.1016/j.fsigen.2017.03.022

[81] ScienceDirect® of Elsevier B.V. Polymerase chain reaction. [Internet]. Available from: http://www.sciencedirect.com/topics/biochemistry-genetics-and-molecular-biology/polymerase-chain-reaction [Accessed: 2017.10.10]

[82] Butler JM. Chapter 4—PCR Amplification: Capabilities and Cautions. In: Advanced Topics in Forensic DNA Typing: Methodology. Academic Press; 2012. pp. 69-97. ISBN: 978-0-12-374513-2. DOI: 10.1016/B978-0-12-374513-2.00004-X

[83] Westen AA, Grol LJ, Harteveld J, et al. Assessment of the stochastic threshold, back- and forward stutter filters and low template techniques for NGM. Forensic Science International. Genetics. 2012;**6**(6):708-715. DOI: 10.1016/j.fsigen.2012.05.001

[84] Gill P, Haned H, Bleka O, et al. Genotyping and interpretation of STR-DNA: Low-template, mixtures and database matches-twenty years of research and development. Forensic Science International. Genetics. 2015;**18**:100-117. DOI: 10.1016/j.fsigen.2015.03.014

[85] Laos R, Thomson JM, Benner SA. DNA polymerases engineered by directed evolution to incorporate non-standard nucleotides. Frontiers in Microbiology. 2014;**5**:565. DOI: 10.3389/fmicb.2014.00565

[86] Grogan DW. Proteins of DNA replication from extreme thermophiles: PCR and beyond. In: Rampelotto P, editor. Biotechnology of Extremophiles: Grand Challenges in Biology and Biotechnology. Vol. 1. Cham: Springer; 2016. pp. 525-538. DOI: 10.1007/978-3-319-13521-2_18

[87] Goodchild J. Conjugates of oligonucleotides and modified oligonucleotides: A review of their synthesis and properties. Bioconjugate Chemistry. 1990;**1**(3):165-187. DOI: 10.1021/bc00003a001

[88] Ballantyne KN, van Oorschot RA, Mitchell RJ. Increased amplification success from forensic samples with locked nucleic acids. Forensic Science International. Genetics. 2011;**5**(4):276-280. DOI: 10.1016/j.fsigen.2010.04.001

[89] Sullivan KM, Pope S, Gill P, Robertson JM. Automated DNA profiling by fluorescent labeling of PCR products. PCR Methods and Applications. 1992;**2**(1):34-40. DOI: 10.1101/gr.2.1.34

[90] GlobalFiler™ Express PCR Amplification Kit USER GUIDE Catalog Numbers 4476609 and 4474665 Publication Number 4477672 Revision E. [Internet]. Available from: https://tools.thermofisher.com/content/sfs/manuals/4477604.pdf [Accessed: 2017.10.10]

[91] Bock JH, Slightom JL. 32P- and fluorescence-labeled DNA sequencing using primers selected from nonamer library. In: Adolph KW, editor. Methods in Molecular Genetics. Vol. 8. Human Molecular Genetics. San Diego, New York, Boston: Academic Press; 1996. pp. 246-257. ISBN: 9780080536415. DOI: 10.1016/S1067-2389(96)80046-X

[92] Shao K, Ding W, Wang F, et al. Emulsion PCR: A high efficient way of PCR amplification of random DNA libraries in aptamer selection. PLoS One. 2011;**6**(9):e24910. DOI: 10.1371/journal.pone.0024910

[93] Kadokami Y, Lewis RV. Membrane bound PCR. Nucleic Acids Research. 1990;**18**(10):3082

[94] Palanisamy R, Connolly AR, Trau M. Considerations of solid-phase DNA amplification. Bioconjugate Chemistry. 2010;**21**(4):690-695. DOI: 10.1021/bc900491s

[95] Tawfik DS, Griffiths AD. Man-made cell-like compartments for molecular evolution. Nature Biotechnology. 1998;**16**:652-656

[96] Kanagal-Shamanna R. Emulsion PCR: Techniques and Applications. In: Luthra R, Singh R, Patel K, editors. Clinical Applications of PCR. Methods in Molecular Biology. Vol. 1392. New York, NY: Humana Press; 2016. pp. 33-42. DOI: 10.1007/978-1-4939-3360-0_4

[97] Mansfield ES, Robertson JM, Vainer M, et al. Analysis of multiplexed short tandem repeat (STR) systems using capillary array electrophoresis. Electrophoresis. 1998;**19**:101-107. DOI: 10.1002/elps.1150190118

[98] Collins PJ, Hennessy LK, Leibelt CS, et al. Developmental validation of a single-tube amplification of the 13 CODIS STR loci, D2S1338, D19S433, and amelogenin: The AmpFlSTR Identifiler PCR Amplification Kit. Journal of Forensic Sciences. 2004;**49**(6): 1265-1277. DOI: 10.1520/JFS2002195

[99] Higuchi R, Fockler C, Dollinger G, Watson R. Kinetic PCR analysis: Real-time monitoring of DNA amplification reactions. Nature Biotechnology. 1993;**11**:1026-1030. DOI: 10.1038/nbt0993-1026

[100] Shi MM, Myrand SP, Bleavins MR, de la Iglesia FA. High throughput genotyping for the detection of a single nucleotide polymorphism in NAD(P)H quinone oxidoreductase (DT diaphorase) using TaqMan probes. Molecular Pathology. 1999;**52**(5):295-299. DOI: http://dx.doi.org/10.1136/mp.52.5.295

[101] Romsos EL, Vallone PM. Rapid PCR of STR markers: Applications to human identification. Forensic Science International. Genetics. 2015;**18**:90-99. DOI: 10.1016/j.fsigen.2015.04.008

[102] Cavanaugh SE et al. Direct PCR amplification of forensic touch and other challenging DNA samples: A review. Forensic Science International. Genetics. 2017;**32**:40-49. DOI: 10.1016/j.fsigen.2017.10.005

[103] Sanger F, Nicklen S, Coulson AR. DNA sequencing with chain-terminating inhibitors. Proceedings of the National Academy of Sciences of the United States of America. 1977; **74**(12):5463-5467

[104] Ronaghi M, Karamohamed S, Pettersson B, et al. Real-time DNA sequencing using detection of pyrophosphate release. Analytical Biochemistry. 1996;**242**(1):84-89. DOI: 10.1006/abio.1996.0432

[105] Timp W, Mirsaidov UM, Wang D, et al. Nanopore sequencing: Electrical measurements of the code of life. IEEE Transactions on Nanotechnology. 2010;**9**(3):281-294. DOI: 10.1109/TNANO.2010.2044418

[106] Børsting C, Morling N. Next generation sequencing and its applications in forensic genetics. Forensic Science International. Genetics. 2015;**18**:78-89. DOI: 10.1016/j.fsigen.2015.02.002

[107] Next-Generation Sequencing – An Overview of the History, Tools, and "Omic" Applications. In: Kulski JK. editor: Next Generation Sequencing—Advances, Applications and Challenges. Intech, 2016. p. 3-60. DOI: 10.5772/61964. Available from: https://www.intechopen.com/books/next-generation-sequencing-advances-applications-and-challenges/next-generation-sequencing-an-overview-of-the-history-tools-and-omic-applications

[108] Butler JM, Coble MD, Vallone PM. STRs vs. SNPs: Thoughts on the future of forensic DNA testing. Forensic Science, Medicine, and Pathology. 2007;**3**(3):200-205. DOI: 10.1007/s12024-007-0018-1

[109] Budowle B, Churchill JD, King JL. Chapter 13—The next state-of-the-art forensic genetics technology: Massively parallel sequencing. In: Amorim A, Budowle B, editors. Handbook of Forensic Genetics: Biodiversity and Heredity in Civil and Criminal Investigation. New Jersey: World Scientific. 2017. p. 249-291. ISBN: 978-1-78634-079-5. DOI: 10.1142/9781786340788_0013

[110] Brion M, Sobrino B, Martinez M, et al. Massive parallel sequencing applied to the molecular autopsy in sudden cardiac death in the young. Forensic Science International. Genetics. 2015;**18**:160-170. DOI: 10.1016/j.fsigen.2015.07.010

[111] Dos Santos Rocha A, de Amorim ISS, Simão TA, et al. High-resolution melting (HRM) of hypervariable mitochondrial DNA regions for forensic science. Journal of Forensic Sciences. 2017. DOI: 10.1111/1556-4029.13552 [Epub ahead of print]

[112] Bruijns B, van Asten A, Tiggelaar R, Gardeniers H. Microfluidic devices for forensic DNA analysis: A review. Caputo D, editor. Biosensors. 2016;**6**(3):41. DOI: 10.3390/bios6030041

[113] Yang J, Brooks C, Estes MD, et al. An integratable microfluidic cartridge for forensic swab samples lysis. Forensic Science International: Genetics. 2014;**8**(1):147-158. DOI: 10.1016/j.fsigen.2013.08.012

[114] Kim YT, Heo HY, Oh SH, et al. Microchip-based forensic short tandem repeat genotyping. Electrophoresis. 2015;**36**(15):1728-1737. DOI: 10.1002/elps.201400477

[115] Han JP, Sun J, Wang L, et al. The optimization of electrophoresis on a glass microfluidic chip and its application in forensic science. Journal of Forensic Sciences. 2017;**62**(6):1603-1612. DOI: 10.1111/1556-4029.13408

[116] Jovanovich S, Bogdan G, Belcinski R, et al. Developmental validation of a fully integrated sample-to-profile rapid human identification system for processing single-source reference buccal samples. Forensic Science International. Genetics. 2015;**16**:181-194. DOI: 10.1016/j.fsigen.2014.12.004

[117] Mapes AA, Kloosterman AD, Poot CJ, van Marion V. Objective data on DNA success rates can aid the selection process of crime samples for analysis by rapid mobile DNA technologies. Forensic Science International. 2016;**264**:28-33. DOI: 10.1016/j.forsciint.2016.03.020

[118] Boiso S, Dalin E, Seidlitz H, et al. RapidHIT for the purpose of stain analyses—An interrupted implementation Forensic Science International: Genetics Supplement Series. 2017;**6**:e589-e590. DOI: http://dx.doi.org/10.1016/j.fsigss.2017.10.002

[119] Primrose SB, Twyman RM. Chapter 2—The organization and structure of genomes. In: Principles of Genome Analysis and Genomics. Blackwell Publishing, 3rd ed. 2003. p. 10-33. ISBN: 978-1-4443-1128-0

[120] Budowle B, Chakraborty R, Giusti AM, et al. Analysis of the VNTR locus D1S80 by the PCR followed by high-resolution PAGE. American Journal of Human Genetics. 1991;**48**: 137-144

[121] Woller J, Furedi S, Padar Z. AMPFLP analysis of the VNTR loci D1S80 and ApoB in Hungary. International Journal of Legal Medicine. 1995;**107**(5):273-274. DOI: 10.1007/BF01245488

[122] Walsh PS, Erlich HA, Higuchi R. Preferential PCR amplification of alleles: Mechanisms and solutions. PCR Methods and Applications. 1992;**1**(4):241-250. DOI: 10.1101/gr.1.4.241

[123] Ellegren H. Microsatellites: Simple sequences with complex evolution. Nature Reviews. Genetics. 2004;**5**(6):435-445. DOI: 10.1038/nrg1348

[124] Urquhart A, Kimpton CP, Downes TJ, Gill P. Variation in short tandem repeat sequences —A survey of twelve microsatellite loci for use as forensic identification markers. International Journal of Legal Medicine. 1994;**107**(1):13-20. DOI: https://doi.org/10.1007/BF01247268

[125] Edwards A, Civitello A, Hammond HA, Caskey CT. DNA typing and genetic mapping with trimeric and tetrameric tandem repeats. American Journal of Human Genetics. 1991;**49**(4):746-756

[126] Van Oorschot RAH, Gutowski SJ, Robinson SL. HUMTH01: Amplification, species specificity, population genetics and forensic applications. International Journal of Legal Medicine. 1994;**107**:121-126. DOI: https://doi.org/10.1007/BF01225598

[127] Furedi S, Woller J, Padar Z. Hungarian population data for the STR systems TH01 and VWA. International Journal of Legal Medicine. 1995;**108**(1):48-49. DOI: https://doi.org/10.1007/BF01845619

[128] Kimpton C, Fisher D, Watson S, et al. Evaluation of an automated DNA profiling system employing multiplex amplification of four tetrameric STR loci. International Journal of Legal Medicine. 1994;**106**(6):302-311. DOI: https://doi.org/10.1007/BF01224776

[129] Füredi S, Budowle B, Woller J, Pádár Z. Hungarian population data on six STR loci—HUMVWFA31, HUMTH01, HUMCSF1PO, HUMFES/FPS, HUMTPOX, and HUMHPRTB —Derived using multiplex PCR amplification and manual typing. International Journal of Legal Medicine. 1996;**109**:100-101. DOI: https://doi.org/10.1007/BF01355526

[130] Füredi S, Angyal M, Kozma Z, et al. Semi-automatic DNA profiling in a Hungarian Romany population using the STR loci HumVWFA31, HumTH01, HumTPOX, and HumCSF1PO. International Journal of Legal Medicine. 1997;**110**(4):184-187. DOI: 10.1007/s004140050064

[131] Butler JM. Chapter 5—Commonly used short tandem repeat markers and commercial kits. In: Forensic DNA Typing: Biology, Technology, and Genetics of STR Markers. 2nd ed. Academic Press; 2005. pp. 85-121. ISBN: 9780080470610

[132] Egyed B, Füredi S, Angyal M, et al. Analysis of eight STR loci in two Hungarian populations. Forensic Science International. 2000;**113**(1–3):25-27. DOI: 10.1016/S0379-0738(00)00191-2

[133] Frank WE, Llewellyn BE, Fish PA, et al. Validation of the AmpFlSTR Profiler Plus PCR amplification kit for use in forensic casework. Journal of Forensic Sciences. 2001;**46**(3): 642-646

[134] Gettings KB, Aponte RA, Vallone PM, Butler JM. STR allele sequence variation: Current knowledge and future issues. Forensic Science International. Genetics. 2015;**18**:118-130. DOI: 10.1016/j.fsigen.2015.06.005

[135] Comey CT, Budowle B. Validation studies on the analysis of the HLA DQ alpha locus using the polymerase chain reaction. Journal of Forensic Sciences. 1991;**36**(6):1633-1648

[136] Budowle B, Woller J, Koons BW, et al. Hungarian population data on seven PCR-based loci. Journal of Forensic Sciences. 1996;**41**(4):667-670. DOI: 10.1520/JFS13975J

[137] Gross AM, Guerrieri RA. HLA DQA1 and Polymarker validations for forensic casework: Standard specimens, reproducibility, and mixed specimens. Journal of Forensic Sciences. 1996;**41**(6):1022-1026

[138] Dimo-Simonin N, Brandt-Casadevall C. Evaluation and usefulness of reverse dot blot DNA-PolyMarker typing in forensic case work. Forensic Science International. 1996; **81**(1):61-72

[139] Syvänen AC, Sajantila A, Lukka M. Identification of individuals by analysis of biallelic DNA markers, using PCR and solid-phase minisequencing. American Journal of Human Genetics. 1993;**52**(1):46-59

[140] Nachman MW, Crowell SL. Estimate of the mutation rate per nucleotide in humans. Genetics. 2000;**156**(1):297-304

[141] Campbell CD, Chong JX, Malig M, et al. Estimating human mutation rate using autozygosity in a founder population. Nature Genetics. 2012;**44**(11):1277-1281. DOI: 10.1038/ng.2418

[142] Sanchez JJ, Phillips C, Børsting C, et al. A multiplex assay with 52 single nucleotide polymorphisms for human identification. Electrophoresis. 2006;**27**(9):1713-1724. DOI: 10.1002/elps.200500671

[143] DLT A, Dennis SE, Salvador JM, et al. Comparison of two massively parallel sequencing platforms using 83 single nucleotide polymorphisms for human identification. Scientific Reports. 2017;**7**:398. DOI: 10.1038/s41598-017-00510-3

[144] Zhang S, Bian Y, Chen A, et al. Developmental validation of a custom panel including 273 SNPs for forensic application using ion torrent PGM. Forensic Science International. Genetics. 2017;**27**:50-57. DOI: 10.1016/j.fsigen.2016.12.003

[145] Gymrek M, Willems T, Reich D, Erlich Y. Interpreting short tandem repeat variations in humans using mutational constraint. Nature Genetics. 2017;**49**(10):1495-1501. DOI: 10.1038/ng.3952

[146] Lang M, Ye Y, Li J, et al. Comprehensive mutation analysis of 53 Y-STR markers in father-son pairs Forensic Science International: Genetics Supplement Series. 2017; DOI: http://dx.doi.org/10.1016/j.fsigss.2017.09.004

[147] Butler JM. Chapter 13—Y-Chromosome DNA Testing. In: Advanced Topics in Forensic DNA Typing: Methodology. Waltham, San Diego: Academic Press; 2012. pp. 371-403. ISBN: 978-0-12-374513-2. DOI: 10.1016/B978-0-12-374513-2.00013-0

[148] Butler JM. Chapter 14—Mitochondrial DNA Analysis. In: Advanced Topics in Forensic DNA Typing: Methodology. Waltham, San Diego: Academic Press; 2012. pp. 405-456. ISBN: 978-0-12-374513-2. DOI: 10.1016/B978-0-12-374513-2.00014-2

[149] Ballantyne KN, Kayser M. Additional Y-STRs in forensics: Why, which, and when. In: Stray JE, editor. Forensic DNA Analysis. Current Practices and Emerging Technologies. Boca Raton, London, New York: CRC Press; 2013. pp. 221-245. ISBN: 978-1-4665-7136-5. DOI: 10.1201/b15361-15

[150] McDonald A, Jones E, Lewis J, O'Rourke P. Y-STR analysis of digital and/or penile penetration cases with no detected spermatozoa. Forensic Science International. Genetics. 2015;**15**:84-89. DOI: 10.1016/j.fsigen.2014.10.015

[151] Hampikian G, Peri G, Lo SS, et al. Case report: Coincidental inclusion in a 17-locus Y-STR mixture, wrongful conviction and exoneration. Forensic Science International. Genetics. 2017;**31**:1-4. DOI: 10.1016/j.fsigen.2017.08.004

[152] Ruitberg CM, Reeder DJ, Butler JM. STRBase: A short tandem repeat DNA database for the human identity testing community. Nucleic Acids Research. 2001;**29**(1):320-322

[153] Willuweit S, Roewer L. Y chromosome haplotype reference database (YHRD): Update. Forensic Science International. Genetics. 2007;**1**(2):83-87. DOI: 10.1016/j.fsigen.2007.01.017

[154] Parson W, Dür A. EMPOP—A forensic mtDNA database. Forensic Science International. Genetics. 2007;**1**(2):88-92. DOI: 10.1016/j.fsigen.2007.01.018

[155] Kayser M. Forensic use of Y-chromosome DNA: A general overview. Human Genetics. 2017;**136**(5):621-635. DOI: 10.1007/s00439-017-1776-9

[156] Shriver MD, Kittles RA. Genetic ancestry and the search for personalized genetic histories. Nature Reviews. Genetics. 2004;**5**(8):611-618. DOI: 10.1038/nrg1405

[157] Calafell F, Larmuseau MHD. The Y chromosome as the most popular marker in genetic genealogy benefits interdisciplinary research. Human Genetics. 2017;**136**(5):559-573. DOI: 10.1007/s00439-016-1740-0

[158] Ermini L, Olivieri C, Rizzi E, et al. Complete mitochondrial genome sequence of the Tyrolean iceman. Current Biology. 2008;**18**(21):1687-1693. DOI: 10.1016/j.cub.2008.09.028

[159] Jobling MA, Tyler-Smith C. Human Y-chromosome variation in the genome-sequencing era. Nature Reviews. Genetics. 2017;**18**(8):485-497. DOI: 10.1038/nrg.2017.36

[160] YHRD – Y-Chromosome Reference Haplotype Database 4.0. [Internet]. Available from: https://yhrd.org [Accessed: 2017.10.10]

[161] Turrina S, Caratti S, Ferrian M, De Leo D. Are rapidly mutating Y-short tandem repeats useful to resolve a lineage? Expanding mutability data on distant male relationships. Transfusion. 2016;**56**(2):533-5388. DOI: 10.1111/trf.13368

[162] Alghafri R, Pajnič Z, Zupanc T, et al. Rapidly mutating Y-STR analyses of compromised forensic samples. International Journal of Legal Medicine. 2017. DOI: 10.1007/s00414-017-1600-z [Epub ahead of print]

[163] Lessig R, Zoledziewska M, Fahr K, et al. Y-SNP-genotyping—A new approach in forensic analysis. Forensic Science International. 2005;**154**(2–3):128-136. DOI: 10.1016/j.forsciint.2004.09.129

[164] Pamjav H, Fehér T, Németh E, Pádár Z. Brief communication: New Y-chromosome binary markers improve phylogenetic resolution within haplogroup R1a1. American Journal of Physical Anthropology. 2012;**149**(4):611-615. DOI: 10.1002/ajpa.22167

[165] Qian X, Hou J, Wang Z, et al. Next generation sequencing plus (NGS+) with Y-chromosomal markers for forensic pedigree searches. Scientific Reports. 2017;**7**(1): 11324. DOI: 10.1038/s41598-017-11955-x

[166] Damas J, Amorim A, Gusmãoet L, et al. InDels in Y chromosome haplogroup definition. Forensic Science International: Genetics Supplement Series. 2011;**3**(1):e178-e179. DOI: 10.1016/j.fsigss.2011.08.089

[167] Wei W, Ayub Q, Chen Y, et al. A calibrated human Y-chromosomal phylogeny based on resequencing. Genome Research. 2013;**23**(2):388-395. DOI: 10.1101/gr.143198.112

[168] Egyed B, Füredi S, Padar Z. Population genetic study in two Transylvanian populations using forensically informative autosomal and Y-chromosomal STR markers. Forensic Science International. 2006;**164**(2–3):257-265. DOI: 10.1016/j.forsciint.2005.10.020

[169] Westen AA, Kraaijenbrink T, Clarisse L, et al. Analysis of 36 Y-STR marker units including a concordance study among 2085 Dutch males. Forensic Science International. Genetics. 2015;**14**:174-181. DOI: 10.1016/j.fsigen.2014.10.012

[170] Gopinath S, Ch Z, Nguyen V, et al. Developmental validation of the Yfiler® plus PCR amplification kit: An enhanced Y-STR multiplex for casework and database applications. Forensic Science International. Genetics. 2016;**24**:164-175. DOI: 10.1016/j.fsigen.2016.07.006

[171] Anderson S, Bankier AT, Barrell BG, et al. Sequence and organization of the human mitochondrial genome. Nature. 1981;**290**(5806):457-465. DOI: 10.1038/290457a0

[172] Coble MD, Just RS, O'Callaghan JE, et al. Single nucleotide polymorphisms over the entire mtDNA genome that increase the power of forensic testing in Caucasians. International Journal of Legal Medicine. 2004;**118**(3):137-146. DOI: 10.1007/s00414-004-0427-6

[173] EMPOP – EDNAP Mitochondrial DNA Population Database, v3/R11. [Internet]. Available from: https://empop.online [Accessed: 2017.10.10]

[174] Gill P, Ivanov PL, Kimpton C, et al. Identification of the remains of the Romanov family by DNA analysis. Nature Genetics. 1994;**6**(2):130-135. DOI: 10.1038/ng0294-130

[175] Coble MD, Loreille OM, Wadhams MJ, et al. Mystery solved: The identification of the two missing Romanov children using DNA analysis. PLoS One. 2009;**4**(3):e4838. DOI: https://doi.org/10.1371/journal.pone.0004838

[176] Li M, Schönberg A, Schaefer M, et al. Detecting heteroplasmy from high-throughput sequencing of complete human mitochondrial DNA genomes. American Journal of Human Genetics. 2010;**87**(2):237-249. DOI: 10.1016/j.ajhg.2010.07.014

[177] Pearce JM. Minding the gap: Frequency of indels in mtDNA control region sequence data and influence on population genetic analyses. Molecular Ecology. 2006;**15**(2):333-341. DOI: 10.1111/j.1365-294X.2005.02781.x

[178] Jun MA, Purcell H, Showalter L, Aagaard KM. Mitochondrial DNA (mtDNA) sequence variation is largely conserved at birth with rare de novo mutations in neonates. American Journal of Obstetrics and Gynecology. 2015;**212**(4):530.e1-530.e8. DOI: 10.1016/j.ajog.2015.02.009

[179] Wilson MR, DiZinno JA, Polanskey D, et al. Validation of mitochondrial DNA sequencing for forensic casework analysis. International Journal of Legal Medicine. 1995;**108**(2):68-74. DOI: https://doi.org/10.1007/BF01369907

[180] Egyed B, Brandstätter A, Irwin JA, et al. Mitochondrial control region sequence variations in the Hungarian population: Analysis of population samples from Hungary and from Transylvania (Romania). Forensic Science International. Genetics. 2007;**1**(2):158-162. DOI: 10.1016/j.fsigen.2007.03.001

[181] Andréasson H, Nilsson M, Styrman H, et al. Forensic mitochondrial coding region analysis for increased discrimination using pyrosequencing technology. Forensic Science International. Genetics. 2007;**1**(1):35-43. DOI: 10.1016/j.fsigen.2006.10.002

[182] Bus MM, Karas O, Allen M. Multiplex pyrosequencing of InDel markers for forensic DNA analysis. Electrophoresis. 2016;**37**(23–24):3039-3045. DOI: 10.1002/elps.201600255

[183] Csősz A, Szécsényi-Nagy A, Csákyová V, et al. Maternal genetic ancestry and legacy of 10(th) century AD Hungarians. Scientific Reports. 2016;**6**:33446. DOI: 10.1038/srep33446

[184] Cocoş R, Schipor S, Hervella M, et al. Genetic affinities among the historical provinces of Romania and Central Europe as revealed by an mtDNA analysis. BMC Genetics. 2017;**18**:20. DOI: 10.1186/s12863-017-0487-5

[185] Fendt L, Zimmermann B, Parson DM, Sequencing W. Strategy for the whole mitochondrial genome resulting in high quality sequences. BMC Genomics. 2009;**10**:139. DOI: 10.1186/1471-2164-10-139

[186] Parson W, Huber G, Moreno L, et al. Massively parallel sequencing of complete mitochondrial genomes from hair shaft samples. Forensic Science International. Genetics. 2015;**15**:8-15. DOI: 10.1016/j.fsigen.2014.11.009

[187] Just RS, Irwin JA, Parson W. Mitochondrial DNA heteroplasmy in the emerging field of massively parallel sequencing. Forensic Science International. Genetics. 2015;**18**:131-139. DOI: 10.1016/j.fsigen.2015.05.003

[188] Irwin JA, Just RS, Parson W. Chapter 14: Massively parallel mitochondrial DNA sequencing in forensic genetics: Principles and opportunities. In: Amorim A, Budowle B, editors. Handbook of Forensic Genetics: Biodiversity and Heredity in Civil and Criminal Investigation. New Jersey: World Scientific; 2017. pp. 293-335. ISBN: 978-1-78634-079-5. DOI: 10.1142/9781786340788_0014

[189] Axler-DiPerte G, Bieber FR, Budimlija ZM, et al. Chapter-18 molecular autopsy. In: Primorac D, Schanfield M. editors. Forensic DNA Applications: An Interdisciplinary Perspective. Boca Raton, London, New York: CRC Press. 2014. p. 453-482. ISBN: 9781466580237

[190] Lombardi R. Genetics and sudden death. Current Opinion in Cardiology. 2013;**28**(3):272-281. DOI: 10.1097/HCO.0b013e32835fb7f3

[191] Lahrouchi N, Behr ER, Bezzina CR. Next-generation sequencing in post-mortem genetic testing of young sudden cardiac death cases. Frontiers in Cardiovascular Medicine. 2016;**3**:13. DOI: 10.3389/fcvm.2016.00013

[192] Sajantila A, Budowle B. Chapter-16: Molecular Autopsy. In: Amorim A, Budowle B, editors. Handbook of Forensic Genetics: Biodiversity and Heredity in Civil and Criminal Investigation. New Jersey: World Scientific; 2017. pp. 377-413. DOI: https://doi.org/10.1142/9781786340788_0016

[193] Bagnall RD, Crompton DE, Semsarian C. Genetic basis of sudden unexpected death in epilepsy. Frontiers in Neurology. 2017;**8**:348. DOI: 10.3389/fneur.2017.00348

[194] Wendt FR, Pathak G, Sajantila A, et al. Global genetic variation of select opiate metabolism genes in self-reported healthy individuals. The Pharmacogenomics Journal. 2017. DOI: 10.1038/tpj.2017.13 [Epub ahead of print]

[195] Seidelmann SB, Smith E, Subrahmanyan L, et al. Application of whole exome sequencing in the clinical diagnosis and management of inherited cardiovascular diseases in adults. Circulation. Cardiovascular Genetics. 2017;**10**(1):e001573. DOI: 10.1161/CIRCGENETICS.116.001573

[196] Butler JM. Chapter 8—DNA databases: Uses and issues. In: Advanced Topics in Forensic DNA Typing: Methodology. Waltham, San Diego: Academic Press; 2012. pp. 213-270. ISBN: 978-0-12-374513-2. DOI: 10.1016/B978-0-12-374513-2.00008-7

[197] Santos F, Machado H. Patterns of exchange of forensic DNA data in the European Union through the Prüm system. Science & Justice. 2017;**57**(4):307-313. DOI: 10.1016/j.scijus.2017.04.001

[198] Jakovski Z, Jankova Ajanovska R, Stankov A, et al. The power of forensic DNA data bases in solving crime cases Forensic Science International: Genetics Supplement Series. 2017;**6**:e275-e276. DOI: http://dx.doi.org/10.1016/j.fsigss.2017.09.085

[199] Bodner M, Bastisch I, Butler JM, et al. Recommendations of the DNA Commission of the International Society for Forensic Genetics (ISFG) on quality control of autosomal short tandem repeat allele frequency databasing (STRidER). Forensic Science International. Genetics. 2016;**24**:97-102. DOI: 10.1016/j.fsigen.2016.06.008

[200] Dembinski GM, Picard CJ. Evaluation of the IrisPlex DNA-based eye color prediction assay in a United States population. Forensic Science International. Genetics. 2014;**9**:111-117. DOI: 10.1016/j.fsigen.2013.12.003

[201] Maroñas O, Phillips C, Söchtig J, et al. Development of a forensic skin colour predictive test. Forensic Science International. Genetics. 2014;**13**:34-44. DOI: 10.1016/j.fsigen.2014.06.017

[202] Phillips C. Forensic genetic analysis of bio-geographical ancestry. Forensic Science International. Genetics. 2015;**18**:49-65. DOI: 10.1016/j.fsigen.2015.05.012

[203] Cheung EYY, Gahan ME, McNevin D. Prediction of biogeographical ancestry from genotype: A comparison of classifiers. International Journal of Legal Medicine. 2017;**131**(4):901-912. DOI: 10.1007/s00414-016-1504-3

[204] Kayser M. Forensic DNA phenotyping: Predicting human appearance from crime scene material for investigative purposes. Forensic Science International. Genetics. 2015;**18**:33-48. DOI: 10.1016/j.fsigen.2015.02.003

[205] Mehta B, Daniel R, Phillips C, McNevin D. Forensically relevant SNaPshot® assays for human DNA SNP analysis: A review. International Journal of Legal Medicine. 2017;**131**(1):21-37. DOI: 10.1007/s00414-016-1490-5

[206] Ambers AD, Churchill JD, King JL, et al. More comprehensive forensic genetic marker analyses for accurate human remains identification using massively parallel DNA sequencing. BMC Genomics. 2016;**17**(Suppl 9):750. DOI: https://doi.org/10.1186/s12864-016-3087-2

[207] Chaitanya L, Pajnič IZ, Walsh S, et al. Bringing colour back after 70 years: Predicting eye and hair colour from skeletal remains of World War II victims using the HIrisPlex system. Forensic Science International. Genetics. 2017;**26**:48-57. DOI: 10.1016/j.fsigen.2016.10.004

[208] Sun Q, Jiang L, Zhang G, et al. Twenty-seven continental ancestry-informative SNP analysis of bone remains to resolve a forensic case. Journal of Forensic Research. 2017;1-3. DOI: http://dx.doi.org/10.1080/20961790.2017.1306431

[209] Li CX, Pakstis AJ, Jiang L, et al. A panel of 74 AISNPs: Improved ancestry inference within eastern Asia. Forensic Science International. Genetics. 2016;**23**:101-110. DOI: 10.1016/j.fsigen.2016.04.002

[210] Pereira V, Mogensen HS, Børsting C, Morling N. Evaluation of the precision ID ancestry panel for crime case work: A SNP typing assay developed for typing of 165 ancestral informative markers. Forensic Science International. Genetics. 2017;**28**:138-145. DOI: 10.1016/j.fsigen.2017.02.013

[211] Wollstein A, Walsh S, Liu F, et al. Novel quantitative pigmentation phenotyping enhances genetic association, epistasis, and prediction of human eye colour. Scientific Reports. 2017;**7**:43359. DOI: 10.1038/srep43359

[212] Jäger AC, Alvarez ML, Davis CP, et al. Developmental validation of the MiSeq FGx forensic genomics system for targeted next generation sequencing in forensic DNA casework and database laboratories. Forensic Science International. Genetics. 2017;**28**: 52-70. DOI: 10.1016/j.fsigen.2017.01.011

[213] Zhu Z, Zhang F, Hu H, et al. Integration of summary data from GWAS and eQTL studies predicts complex trait gene targets. Nature Genetics. 2016;**48**(5):481-487. DOI: 10.1038/ng.3538

[214] Qiao L, Yang Y, Fu P, et al. Genome-wide variants of eurasian facial shape differentiation and a prospective model of DNA based face prediction. bioRxiv:189332. DOI: 10.1101/189332

[215] Freire-Aradas A, Phillips C, Lareu MV. Forensic individual age estimation with DNA: From initial approaches to methylation tests. Journal of Forensic Research. 2017;**29**(2): 121-144

[216] Hong SR, Jung SE, Lee EH, et al. DNA methylation-based age prediction from saliva: High age predictability by combination of 7 CpG markers. Forensic Science International. Genetics. 2017;**29**:118-125. DOI: 10.1016/j.fsigen.2017.04.006

[217] Berkman BE, Shapiro ZE, Eckstein L, Pike ER. The ethics of large-scale genomic research. In: Collmann J, Matei S, editors. Ethical Reasoning in Big Data. Computational Social Sciences. Cham: Springer; 2016. pp. 53-69. ISBN: 978-3-319-28420-0. DOI: 10.1007/978-3-319-28422-4_5

[218] Scudder N, McNevin D, Kelty SF, et al. Massively parallel sequencing and the emergence of forensic genomics: Defining the policy and legal issues for law enforcement. 2017. DOI: 10.1016/j.scijus.2017.10.001 [Epub ahead of print]

[219] Padar Z, Egyed B, Kontadakis K, et al. Canine STR analyses in forensic practice observation of a possible mutation in a dog hair. International Journal of Legal Medicine. 2002;**116**:286-288. DOI: 10.1007/s00414-002-0302-2

[220] Dogan KH, Demirci S. Chapter-5: Livestock-Handling Related Injuries and Deaths. In: Javed K, editor. Livestock Production. New York: InTech; 2012. pp. 81-116. DOI: 10.5772/50834

[221] Halverson JL, Basten C. Forensic DNA identification of animal-derived trace evidence: Tools for linking victims and suspects. Croatian Medical Journal. 2005;**46**(4):598-605

[222] Coyle HM, Lee CL, Lin WY, et al. Forensic botany: Using plant evidence to aid in forensic death investigation. Croatian Medical Journal. 2005;**46**(4):606-612

[223] Rácz E, Könczöl F, Tóth D, et al. PCR-based identification of drowning: Four case reports. International Journal of Legal Medicine. 2016;**130**(5):1303-1307. DOI: 10.1007/s00414-016-1359-7

[224] Kanthaswamy S. Review: Domestic animal forensic genetics—Biological evidence, genetic markers, analytical approaches and challenges. Animal Genetics. 2015;**46**(5):473-484. DOI: 10.1111/age.12335

[225] Menotti-Raymond MA, David VA, O'Brien SJ. Pet cat hair implicates murder suspect. Nature. 1997;**386**(6627):774. DOI: 10.1038/386774a0

[226] Iyengar A, Hadi S. Use of non-human DNA analysis in forensic science: A mini review. Medicine, Science, and the Law. 2014;**54**(1):41-50. DOI: 10.1177/0025802413487522

[227] Arenas M, Pereira F, Oliveira M, et al. Forensic genetics and genomics: Much more than just a human affair. PLoS Genetics. 2017;**13**(9):e1006960. DOI: 10.1371/journal.pgen.100 6960

[228] Budowle B, Murch R, Chakraborty R. Microbial forensics: The next forensic challenge. International Journal of Legal Medicine. 2005;**119**:317-330. DOI: 10.1007/s00414-005-0535-y

[229] Johnson RN, Wilson-Wilde L, Linacre A. Current and future directions of DNA in wildlife forensic science. Forensic Science International. Genetics. 2014;**10**:1-11. DOI: 10.1016/j.fsigen.2013.12.007

[230] Ogden R, Linacre A. Wildlife forensic science: A review of genetic geographic origin assignment. Forensic Science International. Genetics. 2015;**18**:152-159. DOI: 10.1016/j.fsigen.2015.02.008

[231] Zenke P, Egyed B, Pádár Z, Kovács G. Increasing relevance of non-human genetics in Hungarian forensic practice. Forensic Science International: Genetics Supplement Series. 2015;**5**:e412-e413. DOI: 10.1016/j.fsigss.2015.09.100

[232] Beltramo C, Riina MV, Colussi S, et al. Food Control. 2017;**78**:366-373. DOI: 10.1016/j.foodcont.2017.03.006

[233] Staginnus C, Zörntlein S, de Meijer E. A PCR marker linked to a THCA synthase polymorphism is a reliable tool to discriminate potentially THC-rich plants of *Cannabis sativa* L. Journal of Forensic Sciences. 2014;**59**(4):919-926. DOI: 10.1111/1556-4029.12448

[234] Dufresnes C, Jan C, Bienert F, et al. Broad-scale genetic diversity of cannabis for forensic applications. Scali M, editor. PLoS One. 2017;**12**(1):e0170522. DOI: 10.1371/journal.pone.0170522

[235] Schmedes SE, Sajantila A, Budowle B. Expansion of microbial forensics. Journal of Clinical Microbiology. 2016;**54**:1964-1974. DOI: 10.1128/JCM.00046-16

[236] Schmedes SE, Woerner AE, Budowle B. Forensic human identification using skin microbiomes. Applied and Environmental Microbiology. 2017;**83**(22, 12):e01672-17. DOI: 10.1128/AEM.01672-17

[237] Ferri G, Corradini B, Ferrari F, et al. Forensic botany II, DNA barcode for land plants: Which markers after the international agreement? Forensic Science International. Genetics. 2015;**15**:131-136. DOI: 10.1016/j.fsigen.2014.10.005

[238] Wilkinson MJ, Szabo C, Ford CS, et al. Replacing sanger with next generation sequencing to improve coverage and quality of reference DNA barcodes for plants. Scientific Reports. 2017;**7**:46040. DOI: 10.1038/srep46040

[239] De Munnynck K, Van de Voorde W. Forensic approach of fatal dog attacks: A case report and literature review. International Journal of Legal Medicine. 2002;**116**:295-300. DOI: 10.1007/s00414-002-0332-9

[240] Santoro V, Smaldone G, Lozito P, et al. A forensic approach to fatal dog attacks. A case study and review of the literature. Forensic Science International. 2011;**206**(1–3):e37-e42. DOI: 10.1016/j.forsciint.2010.07.026

[241] Bury D, Langlois N, Byard RW. Animal-related fatalities-part I: Characteristic autopsy findings and variable causes of death associated with blunt and sharp trauma. Journal of Forensic Sciences. 2012;**57**:370-374. DOI: 10.1111/j.1556-4029.2011.01921.x

[242] Byard RW. Domestic dogs (*Canis lupus familiaris*) and forensic practice. Forensic Science, Medicine, and Pathology. 2016;**12**:241. DOI: https://doi.org/10.1007/s12024-015-9672-x

[243] Mitsouras K, Faulhaber EA. Saliva as an alternative source of high yield canine genomic DNA for genotyping studies. BMC Research Notes. 2009;**2**:219. DOI: 10.1186/1756-0500-2-219

[244] Yokoyama JS, Erdman CA, Hamilton SP. Array-based whole-genome survey of dog saliva DNA yields high quality SNP data. PLoS One. 2010;**5**(5):e10809. DOI: 10.1371/journal.pone.0010809

[245] Rincon G, Tengvall K, Belanger JM, et al. Comparison of buccal and blood-derived canine DNA, either native or whole genome amplified, for array-based genome-wide association studies. BMC Research Notes. 2011;**4**:226. DOI: 10.1186/1756-0500-4-226

[246] Pádár Z, Egyed B, Kontadakis K, et al. Resolution of parentage in dogs by examination of microsatellites after death of putative sire: Case report. Acta Veterinaria Hungarica. 2001;**49**(3):269-273. DOI: 10.1556/004.49.2001.3.2

[247] Pfeiffer I, Volkel I, Taubert H, Brenig B. Forensic DNA-typing of dog hair: DNA-extraction and PCR amplification. Forensic Science International. 2004;**141**:149-151. DOI: 10.1016/j.forsciint.2004.01.016

[248] Bekaert B, Larmuseau MH, Vanhove MP, et al. Automated DNA extraction of single dog hairs without roots for mitochondrial DNA analysis. Forensic Science International. Genetics. 2012;**6**(2):277-281. DOI: 10.1016/j.fsigen.2011.04.009

[249] Pilli E, Casamassima R, Vai S, et al. Pet fur or fake fur? A forensic approach. Investigative Genetics. 2014;**5**:7. DOI: 10.1186/2041-2223-5-7

[250] Hellmann A, Rohleder U, Schmitter H, et al. STR typing of human telogen hairs: A new approach. International Journal of Legal Medicine. 2001;**114**:269-273

[251] Kun T, Lyons LA, Sacks BN, et al. Developmental validation of Mini-DogFiler for degraded canine DNA. Forensic Science International. Genetics. 2013;**7**(1):151-158

[252] Eichmann C, Parson W. Molecular characterization of the canine mitochondrial DNA control region for forensic applications. International Journal of Legal Medicine. 2007; **121**:411-416. DOI: 10.1007/s00414-006-0143-5

[253] Berger C, Berger B, Parson W. Sequence analysis of the canine mitochondrial DNA control region from shed hair samples in criminal investigations. Methods in Molecular Biology. 2012;**830**:331-348. DOI: 10.1007/978-1-61779-461-2_23

[254] Eichmann C, Berger B, Parson W. A proposed nomenclature for 15 canine-specific polymorphic STR loci for forensic purposes. International Journal of Legal Medicine. 2004;**118**:249-266. DOI: https://doi.org/10.1007/s00414-004-0452-5

[255] Hellmann AP, Rohleder U, Eichmann C, et al. A proposal for standardization in forensic canine DNA typing: Allele nomenclature of six canine-specific STR loci. Journal of Forensic Sciences. 2006;**51**:274-281. DOI: 10.1111/j.1556-4029.2006.00049.x

[256] Kanthaswamy S, Tom BK, Mattila AM, et al. Canine population data generated from a multiplex STR kit for use in forensic casework. Journal of Forensic Sciences. 2009;**54**(4): 829-840. DOI: 10.1111/j.1556-4029.2009.01080.x

[257] Berger B, Berger C, Hecht W, et al. Validation of two canine STR multiplex-assays following the ISFG recommendations for non-human DNA analysis. Forensic Science International. Genetics. 2014;**8**:90-100. DOI: 10.1016/j.fsigen.2013.07.002

[258] Halverson J, Basten C. A PCR multiplex and database for forensic DNA identification of dogs. Journal of Forensic Sciences. 2005;**50**:352-363

[259] Eichmann C, Berger B, Steinlechner M, et al. Estimating the probability of identity in a random dog population using 15 highly polymorphic canine STR markers. Forensic Science International. 2005;**151**:37-44. DOI: 10.1016/j.forsciint.2004.07.002

[260] Van Asch B, Alves C, Gusmao L, et al. A new autosomal STR nineplex for canine identification and parentage testing. Electrophoresis. 2009;**30**(2):417-423. DOI: 10.1002/elps.200800307

[261] Zenke P, Maróti-Agóts A, Padar ZS, et al. Molecular genetic data to evaluate inbreeding in dog populations. — Adatok a kutyaállományok beltenyésztettségének értékeléséhez. Hungarian Veterinary Journal — Magyar Allatorvosok Lapja. 2007;**129**(8):484-489

[262] Zenke P, Maróti-Agóts A, Zs P, et al. Characterization of the WILMS-TF microsatellite marker in Hungarian dog populations. Acta Biologica Hungarica. 2009;**60**(3):329-332. DOI: 10.1556/ABiol.60.2009.3.10

[263] Ganço L, Carvalho M, Serra A, et al. Genetic diversity analysis of 10 STR's loci used for forensic identification in canine hair samples. Forensic Science International: Genetics Supplement Series. 2009;**2**:288-289

[264] Zenke P, Egyed B, Zoldag L, et al. Population genetic study in Hungarian canine populations using forensically informative STR loci. Forensic Science International. Genetics. 2011;**5**(1):e31-e36

[265] Parra D, Garcia D, Mendez S, et al. High mutation rates in canine tetranucleotide microsatellites: Too much risk for genetic compatibility purposes? Open Forensic Science Journal. 2010;**3**:9-13. DOI: 10.2174/1874402801003010009

[266] Periera L, Van Asch B, Amorim A. Standardisation of nomenclature for dog mtDNA D-loop: A prerequisite for launching a *Canis familiaris* database. Forensic Science International. 2004;**141**:99-108. DOI: 10.1016/j.forsciint.2003.12.014

[267] Verscheure S, Backeljau T, Desmyter S. Dog mitochondrial genome sequencing to enhance dog mtDNA discrimination power in forensic casework. Forensic Science International. Genetics. 2014;**12**:60-68. DOI: 10.1016/j.fsigen.2014.05.001

[268] Duleba A, Skonieczna K, Bogdanowicz W, et al. Complete mitochondrial genome database and standardized classification system for *Canis lupus familiaris*. Forensic Science International. Genetics. 2015;**19**:123-129. DOI: 10.1016/j.fsigen.2015.06.014

[269] Oldt R, Ng J, Kanthaswamy S. Chapter-19: The application of forensic animal DNA analysis in criminal and civil investigations. In: Amorim A, Budowle B, editors. Handbook of Forensic Genetics: Biodiversity and Heredity in Civil and Criminal Investigation. New Jersey: World Scientific; 2017. pp. 473-491. DOI: https://doi.org/10.1142/9781786340788_0019

[270] Budowle B, Garofano P, Hellman A, et al. Recommendations for animal DNA forensic and identity testing. International Journal of Legal Medicine. 2005;**119**:295-302. DOI: 10.1007/s00414-005-0545-9

[271] Linacre A, Gusmao L, Hech W, et al. ISFG: Recommendations regarding the use of nonhuman (animal) DNA in forensic genetic investigations. Forensic Science International. Genetics. 2011;**5**:501-505. DOI: 10.1016/j.fsigen.2010.10.017

[272] ENFSI APSTWG. Best Practice Manual for the Application of Molecular Methods for the Forensic Examination of Non-Human Biological Traces. [Internet]. 2015. Available from: http://enfsi.eu/wp-content/uploads/2016/09/8._application_of_molecular_methods_for_the_forensic__examination_of_non-human_biological_traces_0.pdf [Accessed: 2017.10.10]

[273] Bond JW, Weart JR. The effectiveness of trace DNA profiling—A comparison between a U.S. and a U.K. law enforcement jurisdiction. Journal of Forensic Sciences. 2017;**62**(3): 753-760. DOI: 10.1111/1556-4029.13317

[274] ISFG. International Society for Forensic Genetics. Recommendations of the DNA Commission [Internet]. Available from: https://www.isfg.org/Publications/DNA+Commission [Accessed: 2017.10.10]

[275] Padar Z, Nogel M, Kovacs G. Accreditation of forensic laboratories as a part of the 'European Forensic Science 2020' concept in countries of the Visegrad Group. Forensic Science International: Genetics Supplement Series. 2015;**5**:e412-e413. DOI: 10.1016/j.fsigss.2015.09.163

[276] International Organization for Standardization. ISO/IEC 17025:2005. General requirements for the competence of testing and calibration laboratories. [Internet]. Available from: https://www.iso.org/standard/39883.html [Accessed: 2017.10.10]

[277] Alvarez-Cubero MJ, Saiz M, Martínez-García B, et al. Next generation sequencing: An application in forensic sciences? Annals of Human Biology. 2017;**44**(7):581-592. DOI: 10.1080/03014460.2017.1375155

[278] Budowle B, Schmedes SE, Wendt FR. Increasing the reach of forensic genetics with massively parallel sequencing. Forensic Science, Medicine, and Pathology. 2017;**13**(3): 342-349. DOI: 10.1007/s12024-017-9882-5

Chapter 8

Most Common Medico-Legal Autopsy-Related Human and Nonhuman Biological Samples for DNA Analysis

Zsolt Pádár, Petra Zenke and Zsolt Kozma

Additional information is available at the end of the chapter

http://dx.doi.org/10.5772/intechopen.72850

Abstract

The identification and individualization of biological evidences is crucial to actual criminal investigations. In spite of the differences at the national level, all the legal processes attribute particular importance to forensic DNA analysis. However, none of the qualified results from any professional laboratory can produce substantive, valuable evidence with insufficient quality of samples and/or problems with provision of a pristine and controlled environment. The methodology and efficiency of sampling are distinct in case of living persons and in medico-legal autopsy and crime scenes. This chapter is a short overview from the basic introductory information up to ongoing research, and in accordance with constraints on the chapter size, it briefly discusses the important topics of sample collection at medico-legal autopsy for DNA analysis. The content sorts the major types of samples, reviews the common methods of sampling and the potential risk of poor sampling or contamination transfer. The corpses can be more or less degraded, which in special cases (e.g., paraffin embedded tissues, drowned, burning and/or buried cadaver) allow only for analysis of highly degraded samples. The samples can be associated with tissues of a corpse (e.g., blood, soft tissues, bone, tooth, hair) and/or additional extraneous tissues and remains, which are often mixed (e.g., blood, saliva, semen, vaginal fluid, debris of fingernails) on the corpse.

Keywords: medico-legal autopsy, molecular autopsy, autopsy sampling, contamination transfer, forensic genetics

1. Introduction

Medico-legal autopsies usually provide information in connection with violent acts and may provide relevant insight into cases of suicidal, accidental, or unnatural death. The relative volume of autopsies performed can, however, vary from country to country depending on their particular legislation [1]. The classical methodology can nowadays be either partially replaced or may be complemented using modern imaging technologies [2]. The procedures involved in medico-legal autopsies may include the death-scene investigation as well as the ancillary examinations. The demand for better clarifications concerning manner of death have extended the field toward molecular—genetic autopsy [3].

The principal goal of postmortem crime scene examinations and subsequent medico-legal autopsies is to determine, as precisely as possible, the time, cause, and unique circumstances of death. In these proceedings, from the onset of the official crime scene investigation to the conclusion of the professional autopsy performed later in a morgue, close cooperation between the investigation authority and designated forensic medical experts can work to provide the most-accurate answers to these critical questions. The extent of this cooperation must begin by working together at the crime scene through the preservation and evaluation of information gathered during examination and autopsy of the corpse in the morgue. This cooperation is of most importance in cases of violent deaths, where the primary goal is the determination and apprehension of the putative offender as quickly as possible and eventually leading to a subsequent conviction based on irrefutable and verifiable biological evidence.

Connection of a perpetrator to a victim and/or demonstrability of association within the given crime scene, i.e., a proof that a specific act was, or could have been, perpetrated by that individual greatly depends on the amount and quality of physical evidence provided by the authorities. In other words, it depends on the degree of validity of the evidence collected. In most cases, one of the most informative elements of physical evidence is the volume of biological remains/samples that have been secured and preserved at the scene, or during the autopsy and made available for expert examination at a later time. Some of these biological samples may assist in positively associating the perpetrator with the crime scene, while others may confirm the direct participation of an individual in an act of violence which was committed.

These aspects collectively emphasize the absolute necessity of implementing the official procedures as closely as possible in order to effectively procure and preserve contamination-free samples of relevant biological remains. This necessity extends to autopsies as well. The importance of using proper sampling methods during medico-legal procedures cannot be overemphasized. Mitigating the risk of contamination is especially important due to the fact that it may influence expert evaluation and precise interpretation of the results of later laboratory tests. In connection with this, it has also been proven to be important to be able to defend a case against possible legal attacks on the verifiability of these proofs based solely on the method of their procurement, storage, or handling. In regards to contamination, results of an examination can exhibit not only those pertaining to the person or another living being, e.g., animal or plant life, from which the specimen had originally originated, but may also detect postmortem accumulated biological traces acquired through the movement of the corpse, contact during its examination with other people, animals, plants, or other contaminated surfaces, objects, or devices. This is especially relevant in cases of decomposed bodies [4, 5].

The possibility and relevancy of contamination must always be considered. The chance of its occurrence cannot be fully excluded even in the most careful and circumspect proceedings,

http://dx.doi.org/10.5772/intechopen.72850

although we must also note that an insufficiently careful process of decontamination of the body —even on the dissection table—may also result in the elimination of relevant microtraces. With the application of suitable regulations and protocols, the risk can, however, be minimized.

This practice can be important, especially in the cases where a resuscitation attempt was made prior to the crime scene investigation, or when, during the time between the crime scene investigation and the expert autopsy, other individuals may have intervened—for example, manipulation of the corpse during shipment, or there is contact with the pathologists themselves. An increased risk is also present in the case of such practice where the establishment of an isolated infrastructure for the autopsy of a violent death victim in an external location, e.g., graveyard, is either not possible or not entirely suitable, as well as in cases where, for example, in pathology departments or teaching facilities, dissections from multiple cases are performed one after another.

The medico-legal autopsy is one of the first steps in the identification of biological remains. The first, earliest step of characterization of biological evidence in every autopsy room is usually the visual observation with or without the usage of special light sources. For indication of putative nonvictim biological remains, presumptive tests can be applied, followed by an adequate confirmatory test. The proper application of these tests may often result in optimal sampling, however, in the autopsy room, the risk of secondary transfer during manipulation may be elevated [6–9]. The heterogeneity of potential biological evidences even under slightly varying conditions and quality assurance of medico-legal autopsies [10–14], in addition to scientific considerations and practical experience, may also demand a kind of predictive common sense for deliberation during the sampling process to find the optimal result in context of necessary and satisfactory requirements.

2. Most common samples of autopsy for DNA examination, considerations, and characteristics of DNA samplings from victims of violent death

2.1. Victims of sexual assaults (VSA)

In cases of sexual homicide [15–17], in contrast to other forms of homicide—e.g., carried out using a knife or firearm—before the onset of violent death, the offender and the victim are usually in physical contact for a protracted period of time. During this time, even prior to the violent sexual act, the perpetrator attempts to use the true or perceived position of physical power to render the victim unable to act or escape and/or to place them in a state where they cannot defend themselves, as well as to keep them in that state while warding off any attempts at self-defense. In many cases, this is accomplished by covering the mouth and nasal openings —gagging—or grasping of the neck and choking. This series of actions may be accompanied in many cases by stuffing of the external airways and mouth with material. The perpetrator may kiss many parts of the victim's body, may hit the victim, rip their hair as they grasp them, or violently rip off their clothes. The victim may be forcefully penetrated in his/her mouth, anus, or vagina [9], and then, the sexual act may occur involving anal or vaginal penetration—with or without ejaculation [18].

At every stage mentioned above, there is the possibility for the victim and perpetrator to leave biological samples on each other—epithelial cells, saliva, semen, hairs, blood, tears, sweat, urine, or feces. During the victim's attempt at self-protection, the perpetrator most often leaves biological samples of skin, head or body hair and/or saliva on the victim, or under his/her fingernails [19]. The victim may inflict a—possibly bleeding—wound on the perpetrator by biting some parts of his/her body, or biting off, and perhaps even swallowing some piece of a body part. In many cases, the violence is carried out with a partner or in a group, in which case, biological samples from multiple individuals may be found mixed on the victim's body or in some body orifice of the victim, or the victim's self-defense may have been directed at multiple persons. Whatever the case, even in the case of a single attacker, it is unlikely for samples obtainable from the body surface to be of homogeneous origin, while in the case of samples from body orifices, it is almost unavoidable that the biological samples connected to the potential perpetrator be mixed [20]. The careful collection of samples contributes greatly toward increasing the chance for conclusivity of subsequent laboratory tests and/or expert proceedings [21]. Conversely, a lack of care taken in the collection of samples could certainly preclude these results.

Mixed samples found on the victim's clothes, body, or surroundings—animal hairs, plant compounds, earth particles, microorganisms, fungi, etc.—are also preserved from the surroundings where the body was located between the time of the assault and its discovery. The later examination of these can provide important incriminating proof for the criminal procedure [22]. The relevant samples from the perpetrator are usually found in a more homogeneous form on the clothes of the victim than on the body. The corpse may additionally have been washed, denuded, redressed or wrapped, or dragged/transported to a location remote from the site of the crime, or even dismembered.

One of the possible motives for sexual homicide is unfaithfulness, or the suspicion thereof. Consequently, a compulsory part of the autopsy is the examination of the uterus, or in the case where pregnancy is detected, the securing of a biological sample linked to the fetus. This sample may be—depending on the age of the fetus and the postmortem interval—from uterine wall scrapings, placenta, the fetus, or any tissue, organ, blood, umbilical cord, bone, or any other fetal internal organs which contain the DNA of the terminated fetus [23]. In the case of uterine wall scrapings, avoiding the mixture of the mother-fetus samples requires special care, especially in the case of family—genetically related—violence since the mixed genetic profile can influence the statistical interpretation of putative fatherhood [24, 25].

On the basis of the above information, procurement of samples from multiple body surfaces is important—for example, samples from hair, external sexual organs, anus, mouth and nasal orifices, or from the ear region, or from the areas of gripping injury marks on the neck, thigh, or upper arm or internal surfaces may be justified and the relevance of foreign substance remains detected on the skin or fingernails or scratch marks is obvious. Samples may be taken from body cavities—from vaginal and anal cavities, the oral cavity and in some cases from the stomach. Foreign materials used to close off airways or placed in the oral cavity may also carry biological material associated with the perpetrator and, in case of a pregnant victim, the gathering of fetal samples—uterine scrapings, placental or fetal material—is necessary [26].

2.2. Manslaughter (other than VSA)

In the case of non-sexual assault manslaughter cases, contact between the victim and the perpetrator before death either does not occur—e.g., shot from a distance, explosion, poison—or only occurs for a relatively short period. In many cases, it is only indirect, where the perpetrator only goes to the crime location after the event to ensure that the act was successful and that the victim is indeed deceased. Generally, the perpetrator then leans over the victim and/or moves his/her body, during which head and body hairs, sweat, or epithelial cells from the perpetrator's hair, or fingers from where the victim was grasped can be deposited on the body of the victim [27]. In contrast to cases involving sexual violence, we most likely cannot count on discovering more kinds of biological traces or in any greater amounts.

In cases where the violence occurred using some form of equipment, it is necessary—and justified—to preserve samples from items found in, on or around the body, or embedded foreign materials, such as a knife, ammunition, shrapnel or splinters, etc., since it is plausible to attempt identification of the offender from biological samples that remain on these samples [28]. In the case of absence of traces of contact from the perpetrator, samples from the victim's clothing or found in the vicinity—e.g., animal hairs, particular leaves, plant compounds—are of increased importance since some of these may be deposited on the victim postmortem [29–32]. The DNA- or RNA-based examination of these environmental samples may lead to discovery of the primary site of the act in the case where the body has been moved [22, 33, 34]. If physical contact occurs prior to the manslaughter, e.g., a fight or scuffle, then a wider range of biological traces—for example, under the fingernails, epithelial cells at the point of gripping contact, or in the form of sweat, blood or hair—may occur [19, 35, 36]. The quantity of these found is, however, generally nominal.

2.3. Burnt human remains

In the event of home fires, automotive accidents, or disasters such as airplane crashes, industrial disasters accompanied by explosion, or explosive terrorist attacks, the bodies of the deceased have various degrees of burn damage to their tissues and there may also be severe fragmentation, decomposition, and intermixing of the remains of the victims [37, 38]. Rarely, in lucky cases, dental evaluation of intact skulls, examination of special dental implants—possibly containing a serial number, or a serial number on implants from other operations—may lead to the identification of the individual since, in many cases, the classic methods of identification, such as visual recognition, fingerprints, or facial recognition, do not provide usable results. In most cases, it is really only genetic tests which offer any hope of identifying body parts or the deceased individual themselves.

In those cases where the internal organs remain intact under the burnt exterior, genetic-based identification from soft tissue samples does not generally pose a problem. If the strength of the fire has been increased using fire accelerants or perhaps by the combustion of some highly combustible material in the vicinity and the bodies of the deceased have been carbonized, the soft tissue may have been destroyed and the bones severely burnt and more-or-less disintegrated. In this case, genetic analysis may be possible using the lesser burned areas and/or better preserved bones or teeth, although it is important to take into consideration during the sample-gathering process for nuclear or mitochondrial DNA analysis [39–41], the avoidance of areas of potential contamination which could preclude successful genetic examination, e.g., areas burnt with an accelerant, as well as to specifically locate gathering areas which may potentially contain usable information that is difficult or near impossible to visually detect.

Removing contaminants from the path taken by the biological remains from the scene to the laboratory is also essential since, especially fragile, the structurally compromised bone remains can be easily contaminated by contact with other individuals, such as members of the police force officially cooperating in the crime scene investigation, or those people involved in transporting the bones [42].

2.4. Immersed human remains

The identification of drowned bodies—bodies submerged by accident, suicide, or other reasons—such as traffic accident, or postmortem after a murder—that have entered water and sunk, and have decomposed, or are incomplete, is a complex task [43]. In the case of drowning, the typical autopsy findings that aid in determination of cause of death, due to the decomposition process, are mainly absent. In such cases, analysis of those water-dwelling single celled organisms—diatoms and algae—that enter the human bloodstream during drowning is justifiable. For this analysis, it is necessary to obtain samples from, primarily, the lungs or from other organs connected to systemic circulation. Bone marrow and spleen may also be suitable sources of samples for performing diatomic or blue algae specific morphological or genetic examinations [43–46].

Classic methods of identification are significantly limited in the case of bodies discovered that have been soaked for a considerable amount of time, and have started decomposing, have been partly or completely destroyed by possibly boats or driftwood, and are perhaps adipocerous. Visual recognition or facial database-based recognition is impossible, and recognition and identification based on scars from operations or tattoos can be problematic due to the state of the corpse. Examination of the clothing found on the corpse or foreign materials found on its body, for example, a scarf, belt, rope or other object around the neck or extremities, or items—or parts of items—discovered during the autopsy to be trapped inside the body, e.g., bullets, may provide valuable additional information. These may relate to the location that the body entered the water, e.g., the remains of a plant specific to a certain geographical area, or may aid in identification of the individual that used that item. Registered dental records, or serial numbers from special implants may also aid the identification process.

Depending on the length of the postmortem interval (PMI) [47], it would be justified to preserve muscle tissue, blood, hair samples, bone marrow, bone samples, and teeth for later identification of the corpse. These can be obtained using standard techniques during the autopsy. In cases of an aquatic context, the decomposition process may vary [48] and the effectiveness of the tests is significantly affected by the amount of time spent on soaking and in decomposition.

2.5. Highly degraded human bodies or body parts, and human skeletal remains

Recognition and identification of highly fragmented and/or degraded corpses and body parts discovered in advanced stages of decay as described above occur in numerous cases. External environmental conditions, such as climate, weather, and the geographical and geological conditions of the interment, biological components and characteristics of the given location, along with the amount of time the corpse has been exposed to these, play a decisive role in the decomposition processes following onset of death and in the degradation of the nuDNA and mtDNA contents of biological tissues. Due to long PMI, or the corpse being only partial, parts of or even all of it may have experienced significant damage, such as burning, explosion or chemical effects. The affected human soft tissues may be significantly degraded; however, bone and tooth samples can be subjected to and withstand harsher environmental conditions, e.g. ,exposed—burial, water immersion, and still produce varying levels of preservation [37, 49].

Human bones provide a relatively isolated and protected environment and can retain DNA for a long time without significant degradation, i.e., within bone cells, osteocytes, and those cells involved in rebuilding bones, osteoblasts and osteoclasts. The reason for this is that environmental effects—be it degrading enzymes, microorganisms, or ultraviolet rays—are not able to directly damage the DNA contained in the bone. Additionally, the material of the bone has a relatively low water content, meaning that the bone cells can easily dry out. In this case, their DNA bonds with the bone's primary building material such as hydroxylapatite crystals, acting as a protective environment, can preserve even larger sections for an extended period of time [36].

While the relatively suitable preservation of skeletal remains, including teeth, originally provided the main possibility for forensic age determination [50–52], the use of DNA-based molecular methods is currently being investigated [53]. Bone and teeth are the most often used human remains for performing identification using DNA analysis; but, in the case of RNA analysis, they can also be useful for determining PMI [49]. DNA can be isolated with varying degrees of success and effectiveness from different bones in the human body. In the case of a relatively short PMI and an intact corpse, tissues other than bone and teeth, such as blood, muscle, bone marrow, and brain matter, may also be sufficient for the performance of successful genetic analysis. Sometimes, there is even the possibility that instrument fragments or bullets [28] that either passed though the bone or embedded within the bone may preserve foreign DNA from the body of that person or animal that the device passed through before entering the victim's body. The examination of this type of mixed sample may be informative in connection with the circumstances surrounding the death. In the process of securing these samples, attention must be paid to specifying the primary and secondary sampling sites, avoiding contamination and standardization of sample storage [42].

2.6. Victims of animal attacks

Interaction and coexistence with animals may result not only in traumatic injuries, but may also have fatal consequences for humans [54–57]. The types of cases regarding a variety of exotic and wild animals as well as livestock or pets span a wide range from sharp force trauma to poisoning [58–63]. Animal attacks on humans occasionally may turn into lethal accidents, but usually the deaths resulted from unwitnessed attacks [63, 64] require medico-legal investigations. Autopsy evidences can determine the cause of death and reconstruct the dynamics of the fatal event in order to confirm that the attack was accidental and to exclude a mimic homicide [57, 63, 65].

In some cases, the cause of death is sharp and semisharp force trauma, which depends not only on the intensity of the trauma but also to a very great extent on the localization of the injury [65]. Animal biting wounds often permit a reconstruction of the perpetrator's teeth, but postmortem animal depredation may also cause such a bite pattern, which may initially suggest criminal assault [65], especially when animals, e.g., dogs, are enclosed in a home with a corpse [66–68]. Although bite marks can be discriminated from other traumas, bite mark analysis sometimes requires multidisciplinary approaches and should involve different forensic professionals [61, 69].

Although there are a large range of animals that have been involved in attacks on humans, pet dog attacks are relatively the most frequent type of case in medico-legal practice. Ordinarily, the injuries and consequences are related to the vulnerability of the victims, and children, the elderly, and disabled persons have the highest mortality rates [70]. Sometimes the victims of dog attacks are found naked, which can mimic a sexual assault rather than a dog mauling [61, 64]. Similarly to other violence cases, external examination of the corpse can reveal not only the relevant injuries, but also biological traces regarding to a putative perpetrator. Saliva or bitten material from biting area and animal hairs including those from the victims' clothing can be collected for DNA typing [64].

2.7. Collection devices and paraffin embedded tissues

Numerous relevant biological traces may be located on, or spread over the victim's body or in some body orifice. Naked-eye visual recognition and predictive identification of these potentially relevant—albeit in very minute quantity—remains might not be trivial and may require additional tools for preliminary tests. Inadequate or unnecessary sampling might be avoided through merely the technical application of non-invasive detection systems, such as special light sources, and the competence and professional expertise by the person doing the collecting, however, an all-encompassing combination of applied proficiency and practical common sense is necessary as well. Some methods can adversely affect the quality of, or reduce the quantity of retrieved DNA, while others may not pose a risk [71–78].

The application of a secondary transfer surface as a swab is a widely used and preferred protocol [26, 79–82]; however, taping—tape-lifting or stubbing—can be applied alternatively [83–85] for collection of even the epithelial cells of putative offender left on the victim's skin. Various types of swabs and tape are used [84, 86–89]. Retrieval of DNA depends on the sampling force—e.g., the pressure and actuation of the swab and contact intensity of adhesives—at the targeted area of devices and body, but may only partially pick up the available sample. This amount can be increased with multiple and coextracted swabs. In fact, the type of the biological material as well as the ratio of sampling area to the actual area of the deposit of relevant targeted remains, or interaction between victim's cells can influence the amount and mix of samples [89–91]. All this is relevant, even if the secondary transfer material is a liquid (buffer) in a device [92, 93].

Although the contributing sources of DNA can be slightly modified with the careful, deliberate application of secondary devices, the majority of sample profiles usually can be obtained from the victim without trace component separation [82]. Molecular autopsy methods such as laser-capture microdissection (LCM) [94–97], flow cytometry, fluorescence (FACS) or magnetic (MACS) activated cell sorting methodologies [98–101] or alternatives [102–104] are fields where ongoing research is ensuring the potential to enhance the generation of single source genetic profiles of desired target DNA from cellular mixtures obtained by the initial collection device. Recent advances may provide a successful method for the separation of cellular mixtures of small numbers of cells [105], but complete separation of different cells with same morphology and gender origin seems to be a challenge that is still to be adequately addressed [98, 102].

The analysis of formalin-fixed, paraffin-embedded (FFPE) tissue can be essential when the legal process requires retrospective studies, for example, in criminal paternity testing, or cases of sudden unexplained death, or the paraffin blocks are the last and only option, e.g., identification of an unknown body, or for the purpose of determining a genetic profile [106–108], or even the cause and/or manner of death [109]. Formalin fixation process and subsequent storage is a perfect preservative for maintaining the integrity of tissues after death, but it causes crosslinking and degradation-fragmentation of the DNA over time, which prevents molecular PCR analysis and may cause difficulties in genotyping. DNA isolation from FFPE tissue is a decisive step toward a successful examination. Recent advances in technological developments have made generation of genetic information of DNA and RNA from these kinds of challenging samples possible [110–114].

3. Conclusions

Medico-legal autopsies have existed for thousand years, from the primordial period onward. Recently, the wide-ranging scale of procedures, alternative methods, and complementary examinations, such as forensic genetic analysis, are readily available and capable of being carried out for peculiar types of death [115]. Complex issues such as the determination of the postmortem interval, the identification of wound vitality, chronological reconstruction of injuries incurred, or the timing of natural diseases require interdisciplinary approaches and the involvement of multiple specialists, such as the forensic geneticist, among others [116]. In certain cases, the medico-legal autopsy is required by the courts to examine such fatalities in order to determine whether death is attributable to a homicide, suicide, animal attack, or a non-animal related accident, or perhaps due to some unidentified cause [57]. In cases of unknown bodies, skeletons or skeletal remains, as well as for victims of homicides or sexual violence, exemplary professionalism and utilization of appropriate sampling processes are equally important in perfecting the identification of both victims and/or perpetrators. As a primary principle of criminal law, an act must be concluded beyond a reasonable doubt, and a mere technicality, such as the improper preservation of samples or contamination of them, could effectively undermine the entirety of due process and could feasibly prevent a final verdict being made and subsequent sentencing against the true perpetrator of the crime. These aspects demand not only the usage of certified and accredited services and protocols, but also the comprehensive involvement of individual professionals in the field of necroscopic ascertainment—from anatomical dissection to experts in ancillary disciplines, such as the forensic geneticist—to ensure high standards of professional performance [116].

In regards to collection of DNA evidence during autopsy, standard protocols, DNA-free collection devices and appropriate methods of sampling, e.g., swabbings/scrapings/tape-lifting, must of course be taken into consideration along with the collection of trace evidence on the victim's clothing wherever possible. In these instances, application of less invasive methods, such as an alternative light source for identification of body fluids or epithelial cells for potential DNA testing is recommended.

The consideration of, and importance of contamination issues must not be neglected within the autopsy arena. The potential risk of DNA contamination in association with autopsy facilities, equipment, accessories—including impurities of body bags and autopsy tables—must not be ignored, and can be minimized not only by providing the proper protocols and equipment, but more importantly also by the application of personal professionalism [8, 27]. Despite increased attention, and due to the development of more and more sensitive DNA analysis, alternative scenarios are always represented, involving DNA transfer through a secondary person or medium. The minute amount of a few cells or DNA molecules, which may be applicable for amplification, is not recognizable typically in an autopsy environment and is easily transferable between cases [4, 117, 118]. Although methodological developments are continuously making efforts to eliminate the effect of contamination artifacts from the profiling process [119, 120], less appropriate autopsy sampling, incorporating the undetected contamination incidents, can lead to false interpretation within a DNA laboratory [5].

Author details

Zsolt Pádár[1,2]*, Petra Zenke[3] and Zsolt Kozma[1]

*Address all correspondence to: drpadarzsolt@gmail.com

1 Department of Forensic Medicine, Medical School, University of Pécs, Hungary

2 Criminology and Forensic Research Centre, Széchenyi István University, Győr, Hungary

3 Department of Animal Breeding and Genetics, University of Veterinary Medicine, Budapest, Hungary

References

[1] Council of Europe Committee of Ministers. Recommendation no. R (99) 3 of the Committee of Ministers to member states on the harmonization of medico-legal autopsy rules. Forensic Science International. 2000;**111**(1–3):5-29. DOI: https://doi.org/10.1016/S0379-0738(00)00186-9

[2] Bolliger SA, Thali MJ. Imaging and virtual autopsy: Looking back and forward. Philosophical Transactions of the Royal Society of London. Series B, Biological Sciences. 2015; **370**(1674):20140253. DOI: 10.1098/rstb.2014.0253

[3] Torkamani A, Muse ED, Spencer EG, et al. Molecular autopsy for sudden unexpected death. Journal of the American Medical Association. 2016;**316**(14):1492-1494. DOI: 10.1001/jama.2016.11445

[4] Schwark T, Poetsch M, Preusse-Prange A, et al. Phantoms in the mortuary – DNA transfer during autopsies. Forensic Science International 2012;**216**(1–3): 121–126. DOI: 10.1016/j.forsciint.2011.09.006

[5] Kovács G, Padar Z. Misinterpretation of sample contamination in a Hungarian casework. Forensic Science International: Genetics Supplement Series. 2015;**5**:e425-e427. DOI: http://dx.doi.org/10.1016/j.fsigss.2015.09.169

[6] Goray M, Mitchell RJ, van Oorschot RA. Investigation of secondary DNA transfer of skin cells under controlled test conditions. Legal Medicine (Tokyo). 2010;**12**(3):117-120. DOI: 10.1016/j.legalmed.2010.01.003

[7] Wiegand P, Heimbold C, Klein R, et al. Transfer of biological stains from different surfaces. International Journal of Legal Medicine 2011;**125**:727-731. DOI: 10.1007/s00414-010-0424-x

[8] Szkuta B, Harvey ML, Ballantyne KN, et al. DNA transfer by examination tools – A risk for forensic casework? Forensic Science International. Genetics. 2015;**16**:246-254. DOI: 10.1016/j.fsigen.2015.02.004

[9] Balk C. Reducing contamination in forensic science. Themis: Research Journal of Justice Studies and Forensic Science. 2015;**3**(1):Art. 12. Available from: http://scholarworks.sjsu.edu/themis/vol3/iss1/12 [Accessed: Oct 10, 2017]

[10] Kotabag RB, Charati SC, Jayachandar D. Clinical autopsy vs medicolegal autopsy. Medical Journal Armed Forces India. 2005;**61**(3):258-263. DOI: 10.1016/S0377-1237(05)80169-8

[11] Lunetta P, Lounamaa A, Sihvonen S. Surveillance of injury-related deaths: Medicolegal autopsy rates and trends in Finland. Injury Prevention. 2007;**13**(4):282-284. DOI: 10.1136/ip.2006.012922

[12] Van den Tweel JG, Wittekind C. The medical autopsy as quality assurance tool in clinical medicine: Dreams and realities. Virchows Archiv. 2016;**468**:75-81. DOI: 10.1007/s00428-015-1833-5

[13] Kelsall D, Bowes MJ. No standards: Medicolegal investigation of deaths. Canadian Medical Association Journal. 2016;**188**(3):169. DOI: 10.1503/cmaj.160041

[14] Conran RM. Medicolegal issues and the autopsy. Medscape. [Internet]. Available from: https://emedicine.medscape.com/article/1975045-overview#showall [Accessed: Oct 10, 2017]

[15] Youssef N, Wiem BA, Zouheir H, Samir M. Sexual homicide committed by a family member: Report of two cases and discussion of its motivation factors. Journal of Forensic Medicine. 2016;**2**:112. DOI: 10.4172/2472-1026.1000112

[16] Mahanta P. Case report rape, sodomy and murder of a minor girl. Journal of Indian Academy of Forensic Medicine 2012;**34**(4):358-360. Available from: http://medind.nic.in/jal/t12/i4/jalt12i4p358.pdf [Accessed: Oct 10, 2017]

[17] Sinha NK, RoyChowdhury UB, Das DC, et al. Sexual abuse and murder of a minor girl: A case study. Indian Journal of Forensic and Community Medicine. 2015;**2**(4):251-254. DOI: 10.5958/2394-6776.2015.00011.9

[18] Casey DG, Domijan K, MacNeill S, et al. The persistence of sperm and the development of time since intercourse (TSI) guidelines in sexual assault cases at forensic science Ireland, Dublin, Ireland. Journal of Forensic Sciences 2017;**62**(3):585-592. DOI: 10.1111/1556-4029.13325

[19] Wiegand P, Bajanowski T, Brinkmann B. DNA typing of debris from fingernails. International Journal of Legal Medicine. 1993;**106**:81-83. DOI: 10.1007/BF01225045

[20] Gingras F, Paquet C, Bazinet M, et al. Biological and DNA evidence in 1000 sexual assault cases. Forensic Science International: Genetics Supplement Series 2009;**2**(1):138-140. DOI: http://dx.doi.org/10.1016/j.fsigss.2009.09.006

[21] McGregor MJ, Du Mont J, Myhr TL. Sexual assault forensic medical examination: Is evidence related to successful prosecution? Annals of Emergency Medicine. 2002;**39**(6):639-647. DOI: http://dx.doi.org/10.1067/mem.2002.123694

[22] Yoon CK. Botanical witness for the prosecution. Science 1993;**260**(5110):894-895. DOI: 10.1126/science.8493521

[23] Csete K, Zs B, Varga T. Prenatal and newborn paternity testing with DNA analysis. Forensic Science International Supplement Series. 2005;**147**:S57-S60. DOI: 10.1016/j.forsciint.2004.09.101

[24] Lee JC, Tsai LC, Chu PC, et al. The risk of false inclusion of a relative in parentage testing – An in silico population study. Croatian Medical Journal. 2013;**54**(3):257-262. DOI: 10.3325/cmj.2013.54.257

[25] Green PJ, Mortera J. Paternity testing and other inference about relationships from DNA mixtures. Forensic Science International. Genetics. 2017;**28**:128-137. DOI: 10.1016/j.fsigen.2017.02.001

[26] Magalhães T, Dinis-Oliveira RJ, Silva B, et al. Biological evidence management for DNA analysis in cases of sexual assault. ScientificWorldJournal. 2015;**2015**:365674. DOI: 10.1155/2015/365674

[27] Prahlow JA, Cameron T, Arendt A, et al. DNA testing in homicide investigations. Medicine, Science, and the Law 2017;**57**(4):179-191. DOI: 10.1177/0025802417721790

[28] Dieltjes P, Mieremet R, Zuniga S, et al. A sensitive method to extract DNA from biological traces present on ammunition for the purpose of genetic profiling. International Journal of Legal Medicine. 2011;**125**(4):597-602. DOI: 10.1007/s00414-010-0454-4

[29] Menotti-Raymond MA, David VA, O'Brien SJ. Pet cat hair implicates murder suspect. Nature. 1997;**386**(6627):774. DOI: 10.1038/386774a0

[30] Halverson JL, Basten C. Forensic DNA identification of animal-derived trace evidence: Tools for linking victims and suspects. Croatian Medical Journal. 2005;**46**(4):598-605

[31] Coyle HM, Lee CL, Lin WY, et al. Forensic botany: Using plant evidence to aid in forensic death investigation. Croatian Medical Journal. 2005;**46**(4):606-612

[32] Craft KJ, Owens JD, Ashley MV. Application of plant DNA markers in forensic botany: Genetic comparison of Quercus evidence leaves to crime scene trees using microsatellites. Forensic Science International 2007;**165**(1):64-70. DOI: 10.1016/j.forsciint.2006.03.002

[33] Wesselink M, Kuiper I. Species identification of botanical trace evidence using molecular markers. Forensic Science International: Genetics Supplement Series. 2008;**1**(1):630-632. DOI: https://doi.org/10.1016/j.fsigss.2007.10.211

[34] Bell KL, Burgess KS, Okamoto KC, et al. Review and future prospects for DNA barcoding methods in forensic palynology. Forensic Science International. Genetics. 2016;**21**:110-116. DOI: 10.1016/j.fsigen.2015.12.010

[35] Padar Z, Barta A, Egyed B, et al. Hungarian experience of examination of the fingernails in violent crime. In: Sensabaugh GF, Lincoln P, Olaisen B, editors. Progress in Forensic Genetics 8: Proceedings of the 18th International ISFH Congress, San Francisco, CA. USA, 17–21 August 1999. Amsterdam, Lausanne, New York et al.: Elsevier (ICS 1193); 2000. pp. 492-494. ISBN: 978-0444503039

[36] Parsons TJ, Weedn VW. Preservation and recovery of DNA in postmortem specimens and trace samples. In: Haglund W, Sorg M, editors. Advances in Forensic Taphonomy: The Fate of Human Remains. New York: CPR Press; 1996. pp. 109-138. DOI: 10.1201/9781439821923.ch7

[37] Imaizumi K. Forensic investigation of burnt human remains. Research and Reports in Forensic Medical Science. 2005;**5**:67-74. DOI: https://doi.org/10.2147/RRFMS.S75141

[38] Ziętkiewicz E, Witt M, Daca P, et al. Current genetic methodologies in the identification of disaster victims and in forensic analysis. Journal of Applied Genetics 2012;**53**(1):41-60. DOI: 10.1007/s13353-011-0068-7

[39] Schwark T, Heinrich A, Preusse-Prange A, von Wurmb-Schwark N. Reliable genetic identification of burnt human remains. Forensic Science International. Genetics. 2011; **5**(5):393-399. DOI: 10.1016/j.fsigen.2010.08.008

[40] Li R, Klempner S. The effect of an enzymatic bone processing method on short tandem repeat profiling of challenged bone specimens. Legal Medicine (Tokyo). 2013;**15**(4):171-176. DOI: 10.1016/j.legalmed.2012.12.002

[41] Zupanič Pajnič I, Debska M, Gornjak Pogorelc B, et al. Highly efficient automated extraction of DNA from old and contemporary skeletal remains. Journal of Forensic and Legal Medicine 2016;**37**:78-86. DOI: 10.1016/j.jflm.2015.11.001

[42] Standard Operating Procedure for Sampling Bone and Tooth Specimens From Human Remains for DNA Testing at the ICMP, International Commision of Missing Persons:

ICMP.SOP.AA.136.2.doc, Sarajevo, February 16, 2015. [Internet]. Available from: https://www.icmp.int/?resources=standard-operating-procedure-for-sampling-bone-and-tooth-specimens-from-human-remains-for-dna-testing-at-the-icmp-2 [Accessed: Oct 10, 2017]

[43] Delabarde T, Keyser C, Tracqui A, et al. The potential of forensic analysis on human bones found in riverine environment. Forensic Science International 2013;**228**(1–3):e1-e5. DOI: 10.1016/j.forsciint.2013.03.019

[44] Brenda LW, editor. Handbook of Autopsy Practice, 4th ed. Humana Press; 2010. pp. 272-274. DOI: 10.1007/978-1-59745-127-7. ISBN: 978-1-58829-841-6

[45] Rácz E, Könczöl F, Tóth D, et al. PCR-based identification of drowning: Four case reports. International Journal of Legal Medicine. 2016;**130**(5):1303-1307. DOI: 10.1007/s00414-016-1359-7

[46] Takeichi T, Kitamura O. Detection of diatom in formalin-fixed tissue by proteinase K digestion. Forensic Science International. 2009;**190**(1–3):19-23. DOI: 10.1016/j.forsciint.2009.05.005

[47] Dickson GC, Poulter RT, Maas EW, et al. Marine bacterial succession as a potential indicator of postmortem submersion interval. Forensic Science International. 2011;**209**(1–3):1-10. DOI: 10.1016/j.forsciint.2010.10.016

[48] Borde YM, Tonnany MB, Champod C. A study on the effects of immersion in river water and seawater on blood, saliva, and sperm placed on objects mimicking crime scene exhibits. Canadian Society of Forensic Science Journal. 2008;**41**(3):149-163. DOI: 10.1080/00085030.2008.10757172

[49] Poór VS, Lukács D, Nagy T, et al. The rate of RNA degradation in human dental pulp reveals post-mortem interval. International Journal of Legal Medicine 2016;**130**:615-619. DOI: 10.1007/s00414-015-1295-y

[50] Cardoso HFV, Spake L, Liversidge HM. A reappraisal of developing permanent tooth length as an estimate of age in human immature skeletal remains. Journal of Forensic Sciences. 2016;**61**(5):1180-1189. DOI: 10.1111/1556-4029.13120

[51] Cardoso HFV, Vandergugten JM, Humphrey LT. Age estimation of immature human skeletal remains from the metaphyseal and epiphyseal widths of the long bones in the post-natal period. American Journal of Physical Anthropology. 2017;**162**(1):19-35. DOI: 10.1002/ajpa.23081

[52] Cardoso HFV, Spake L, Humphrey LT. Age estimation of immature human skeletal remains from the dimensions of the girdle bones in the postnatal period. American Journal of Physical Anthropology. 2017;**163**(4):772-783. DOI: 10.1002/ajpa.23248

[53] Freire-Aradas A, Phillips C, Lareu MV. Forensic individual age estimation with DNA: From initial approaches to methylation tests. Forensic Science Review 2017;**29**(2):121-144

[54] Bury D, Langlois N, Byard RW. Animal-related fatalities-part I: Characteristic autopsy findings and variable causes of death associated with blunt and sharp trauma. Journal of Forensic Sciences. 2012;**57**:370-374. DOI: 10.1111/j.1556-4029.2011.01921.x

[55] Bury D, Langlois N, Byard RW. Animal-related fatalities-part II: Characteristic autopsy findings and variable causes of death associated with envenomation, poisoning, anaphylaxis, asphyxiation, and sepsis. Journal of Forensic Sciences. 2012;**57**:375-380. DOI: 10.1111/j.1556-4029.2011.01932.x

[56] Dogan KH, Demirci S. Chapter – 5: Livestock-handling related injuries and deaths. In: Javed K, editor. Livestock Production. New York: InTech; 2012. pp. 81-116. DOI: 10.5772/50834

[57] Da Broi U, Moreschi C, Fanzutto A, et al. Medico-legal implications of traumatic fatalities related to animal husbandry. Contemporary Engineering Sciences. 2015;**8**(25):1153-1162. HIKARI Ltd. Available from: www.m-hikari.com. DOI: http://dx.doi.org/10.12988/ces.2015.56173

[58] Wolf BC, Harding BE. Fatalities due to indigenous and exotic species in Florida. Journal of Forensic Sciences. 2014;**59**(1):155-160. DOI: 10.1111/1556-4029.12261

[59] Škavić P, Šprem N, Kostelić A. Fatal injury caused by a Ram (Ovis Aries) attack. Journal of Forensic Sciences. 2015;**60**(5):1380-1382. DOI: 10.1111/1556-4029.12813

[60] Tsung AH, Allen BR. A 51-year-old woman crushed by an elephant trunk. Wilderness & Environmental Medicine. 2015;**26**(1):54-58. DOI: 10.1016/j.wem.2014.07.006

[61] Fonseca GM, Mora E, Lucena J, et al. Forensic studies of dog attacks on humans: A focus on bite mark analysis. Research and Reports in Forensic Medical Science 2015;**5**:39-51. DOI: https://doi.org/10.2147/RRFMS.S92068

[62] Szleszkowski Ł, Thannhäuser A, Jurek T. Compound mechanism of fatal neck injury: A case report of a tiger attack in a zoo. Forensic Science International. 2017;**277**:e16-e20. DOI: 10.1016/j.forsciint.2017.05.011

[63] Gudmannsson P, Berge J, Druid H, et al. A unique fatal moose attack mimicking homicide. Journal of Forensic Sciences. 2017. DOI: 10.1111/1556-4029.13579 [Epub ahead of print]

[64] Padar Z, Egyed B, Kontadakis K, et al. Canine STR analyses in forensic practice observation of a possible mutation in a dog hair. International Journal of Legal Medicine 2002; **116**:286-288. DOI: 10.1007/s00414-002-0302-2

[65] Dettmeyer RB, Verhoff MA, Schütz HF. Pointed, sharp, and semi-sharp force trauma. In: Forensic Medicine: Fundamentals and Perspectives. Spring. 2014. pp. 135-153. ISBN: 978-3-642-38818-7. DOI: 10.1007/978-3-642-38818-7

[66] Verzeletti A, Cortellini V, Vassalini M. Post-mortem injuries by a dog: A case report. Journal of Forensic and Legal Medicine. 2010;**17**(4):216-219. DOI: 10.1016/j.jflm.2009.12.011

[67] Hernández-Carrasco M, Pisani JMA, Scarso-Giaconi F, Fonseca GM. Indoor postmortem mutilation by dogs: Confusion, contradictions, and needs from the perspective of the forensic veterinarian medicine. Journal of Veterinary Behavior: Clinical Applications and Research. 2016;**15**:56-60. DOI: https://doi.org/10.1016/j.jveb.2016.08.074

[68] Omond KJ, Winskog C, Cala A, Byard RW. Neonatal limb amputation-an unusual form of postmortem canine predation. Journal of Forensic Sciences. 2017;**62**(4):937-939. DOI: 10.1111/1556-4029.13378

[69] Salem NH, Belhadj M, Aissaoui A, et al. Multidisciplinary approach to fatal dog attacks: A forensic case study. Journal of Forensic and Legal Medicine 2013;**20**(6):763-766. DOI: 10.1016/j.jflm.2013.04.015

[70] De Munnynck K, Van de Voorde W. Forensic approach of fatal dog attacks: A case report and literature review. International Journal of Legal Medicine. 2002;**116**:295-300. DOI: 10.1007/s00414-002-0332-9

[71] Stoilovic M. Detection of semen and blood stains using Polilight as a light source. Forensic Science International. 1991;**51**:289-296. DOI: 10.1016/0379-0738(91)90194-N

[72] Gross AM, Harris KA, Kaldun GL. The effect of luminol on presumptive tests and DNA analysis using the polymerase chain reaction. Journal of Forensic Sciences. 1999;**44**(4): 837-840. DOI: 10.1520/JFS14561J

[73] Forensic Science in North Carolina. Noureddine M. Forensic Tests for Semen: What You Should Know. [Internet]. 2011. Available from: https://ncforensics.wordpress.com/2011/10/19/forensic-tests-for-semen-what-you-should-know/ [Accessed: Oct 10, 2017]

[74] Forensic Science in North Carolina. Noureddine M. Forensic Tests for Saliva: What You Should Know. [Internet]. 2011. Available from: https://ncforensics.wordpress.com/2011/10/19/forensic-tests-for-semen-what-you-should-know/ [Accessed: Oct 10, 2017]

[75] De Almeida JP, Glesse N, Bonorino C. Effect of presumptive tests reagents on human blood confirmatory tests and DNA analysis using real time polymerase chain reaction. Forensic Science International. 2011 Mar 20;**206**(1–3):58-61. DOI: 10.1016/j.forsciint.2010.06.017

[76] Vandenberg N, van Oorschot RAH. The use of Polilight in the detection of seminal fluid, saliva and bloodstains and comparison with conventional chemical-based screening tests. Journal of Forensic Sciences. 2006;**51**:361-370. DOI: 10.1111/j.1556-4029.2006.00065.x

[77] Vandewoestyne M, Lepez T, Van Hoofstat D, Deforce D. Evaluation of a visualization assay for blood on forensic evidence. Journal of Forensic Sciences. 2015;**60**(3):707-711. DOI: 10.1111/1556-4029.12720

[78] Donachie GE, Dawnay N, Ahmed R, et al. Assessing the impact of common forensic presumptive tests on the ability to obtain results using a novel rapid DNA platform. Forensic Science International. Genetics 2015;**17**:87-90. DOI: 10.1016/j.fsigen.2015.04.003

[79] Sweet D, Lorente M, Lorente JA, et al. An improved method to recover saliva from human skin: The double swab technique. Journal of Forensic Sciences. 1997;**42**:320-322

[80] Hochmeister M, Rudin, Meier R, et al. A foldable cardboard box for drying and storage of by cotton swab collected biological samples. Archiv für Kriminologie 1997;**200**(3–4): 113-120

[81] Pang BCM, Cheung BKK. Double swab technique for collecting touched evidence. Legal Medicine. 2007;**9**:181-184. DOI: 10.1016/j.legalmed.2006.12.003

[82] Adamowicz MS, Stasulli DM, Sobestanovich EM, Bille TW. Evaluation of methods to improve the extraction and recovery of DNA from cotton swabs for forensic analysis. PLoS One. 2014;**9**(12):e116351. DOI: https://doi.org/10.1371/journal.pone.0116351

[83] De Bruin KG, Verheij SM, Veenhoven M, Sijen T. Comparison of stubbing and the double swab method for collecting offender epithelial material from a victim's skin. Forensic Science International. Genetics. 2012;**6**(2):219-223. DOI: 10.1016/j.fsigen.2011.04.019

[84] Verdon TJ, Mitchell RJ, van Oorschot RA. Evaluation of tapelifting as a collection method for touch DNA. Forensic Science International. Genetics. 2014;**8**(1):179-186. DOI: 10.1016/j.fsigen.2013.09.005

[85] Forsberg C, Jansson L, Ansell R, Hedman J. High-throughput DNA extraction of forensic adhesive tapes. Forensic Science International. Genetics. 2016;**24**:158-163. DOI: 10.1016/j.fsigen.2016.06.004

[86] Hansson O, Finnebraaten M, Knutsen Heitmann I, et al. Trace DNA collection – Performance of minitape and three different swabs. Forensic Science International: Genetics Supplement Series 2009;**2**:189-190. DOI: 10.1016/j.fsigss.2009.08.098

[87] Verdon TJ, Mitchell RJ, van Oorschot RA. Swabs as DNA collection devices for sampling different biological materials from different substrates. Journal of Forensic Sciences. 2014;**59**(4):1080-1089. DOI: 10.1111/1556-4029.12427

[88] Verdon TJ, Mitchell RJ, van Oorschot RA. Preliminary investigation of differential tapelifting for sampling forensically relevant layered deposits. Legal Medicine (Tokyo). 2015;**17**(6):553-559. DOI: 10.1016/j.legalmed.2015.07.002

[89] Plaza DT, Mealy JL, Lane JN, et al. Nondestructive biological evidence collection with alternative swabs and adhesive lifters. Journal of Forensic Sciences. 2016;**61**(2):485-488. DOI: 10.1111/1556-4029.12980

[90] Van Oorschot RAH, Ballantyne KN, Mitchell RJ. Forensic trace DNA: A review. Investigative Genetics. 2010;**1**:14. DOI: 10.1186/2041-2223-1-14

[91] Van Oorschot RAH, Verdon TJ, Ballantyne KN. Collection of samples for DNA analysis. In: Goodwin W, editor. Forensic DNA Typing Protocols. Methods in Molecular Biology. Vol. 1420. New York: Humana Press. 2016. DOI: https://doi.org/10.1007/978-1-4939-3597-0_1

[92] Hedman J, Agren J, Ansel R. Crime scene DNA sampling by wet-vacuum applying M-Vac. Forensic Science International: Genetics Supplement Series. 2015;**5**:e89-e90. DOI: http://dx.doi.org/10.1016/j.fsigss.2015.09.036

[93] Williams S, Panacek E, Green W, et al. Recovery of salivary DNA from the skin after showering. Forensic Science, Medicine, and Pathology 2015;**11**(1):29–34. DOI: 10.1007/s12024-014-9635-7

[94] Espina V, Milia J, Wu G, et al. Laser capture microdissection. In: Taatjes DJ, Mossman BT, editors. Cell Imaging Techniques. Methods in Molecular Biology. Vol. 319. Totowa: Humana Press; 2006. pp. 213-229. DOI: https://doi.org/10.1007/978-1-59259-993-6_10

[95] Anslinger K, Bayer B, Mack B, Eisenmenger W. Sex-specific fluorescent labelling of cells for laser microdissection and DNA profiling. International Journal of Legal Medicine. 2007;**121**:54-56. DOI: 10.1007/s00414-005-0065-7

[96] Vandewoestyne M, Deforce D. Laser capture microdissection for forensic DNA analysis. Forensic Science International: Genetics Supplement Series. 2011;**3**(1):e117-e118. DOI: http://dx.doi.org/10.1016/j.fsigss.2011.08.058

[97] Zhang L, Ding M, Pang H, et al. Mitochondrial DNA typing of laser-captured single sperm cells to differentiate individuals in a mixed semen stain. Electrophoresis 2016; **37**(15–16):2273-2277. DOI: 10.1002/elps.201600009

[98] Rieseberg M, Kasper C, Readon KF, Scheper T. Flow cytometry in biotechnology. Applied Microbiology and Biotechnology. 2001;**56**:350-360. DOI: 10.1007/s002530100673

[99] Verdon, TJ. Mitchell RJ, Chen W, et al. FACS separation of non-compromised forensically relevant biological mixtures. Forensic Science International. Genetics. 2015;**14**:194-200. DOI: 10.1016/j.fsigen.2014.10.019

[100] Xu Y, Xie J, Chen R, et al. Fluorescence- and magnetic-activated cell sorting strategies to separate spermatozoa involving plural contributors from biological mixtures for human identification. Scientific Reports. 2016;**6**:36515. DOI: 10.1038/srep36515

[101] Katherine MP, Stanciu CE, Kwon YJ, et al. Analysis of cellular autofluorescence in touch samples by flow cytometry: Implications for front end separation of trace mixture evidence. Analytical and Bioanalytical Chemistry. 2017;**409**:4167. DOI: https://doi.org/10.1007/s00216-017-0364-0

[102] Schneider C, Müller U, Kilper R, Siebertz B. Low copy number DNA profiling from isolated sperm using the aureka® – Micromanipulation system. Forensic Science International. Genetics. 2012;**6**(4):461-465. DOI: 10.1016/j.fsigen.2011.10.001

[103] Grosjean F, Castella V. A new approach for the separation of spermatozoa from other cell types in forensically relevant samples Forensic Science International: Genetics Supplement Series 2015;**5**:e653-e655. DOI: https://doi.org/10.1016/j.fsigss.2015.10.013

[104] Zhao XC, Wang L, Sun J, et al. Isolating sperm from cell mixtures using magnetic beads coupled with an anti-PH-20 antibody for forensic DNA analysis. PLoS One 2016;**11**(7): e0159401. DOI: 10.1371/journal.pone.0159401

[105] Fontana F, Rapone C, Bregola G, et al. Isolation and genetic analysis of pure cells from forensic biological mixtures: The precision of a digital approach. Forensic Science International. Genetics 2017;**29**:225-241. DOI: 10.1016/j.fsigen.2017.04.023

[106] Zehner R, Lasczkowski G. Paternity-testing on paraffin-embedded abortion tissue: preparation of fetal cells may be indispensable. Journal of Forensic Sciences. 2000;**45**(6):1332-1334. DOI: https://doi.org/10.1520/JFS14891J

[107] Nascimento E, Cerqueira E, Azevedo E, et al. Genotyping of DNA samples under adverse conditions of low copy number – LCN (formolisados tissue samples and embedded in paraffin) Forensic Science International: Genetics Supplement Series 2009; **2**(1):155-156. DOI: http://dx.doi.org/10.1016/j.fsigss.2009.09.019

[108] Reshef A, Barash M, Voskoboinik L, et al. STR typing of formalin-fixed paraffin embedded (FFPE) aborted foetal tissue in criminal paternity cases. Science & Justice. 2011;**51**(1): 19-23. DOI: 10.1016/j.scijus.2010.09.001

[109] Reid KM, Maistry S, Ramesar R, Heathfield LJ. A review of the optimisation of the use of formalin fixed paraffin embedded tissue for molecular analysis in a forensic postmortem setting. Forensic Science International. 2017;**280**:181-187. DOI: 10.1016/j.forsciint.2017.09.020

[110] Baak-Pablo R, Dezentje V, Guchelaar HJ, et al. Genotyping of DNA samples isolated from formalin-fixed paraffin-embedded tissues using Preamplification. Molecular Diagnosis. 2010;**12**(6):746-749. DOI: 10.2353/jmoldx.2010.100047

[111] Okello JB, Zurek J, Devault AM, et al. Comparison of methods in the recovery of nucleic acids from archival formalin-fixed paraffin-embedded autopsy tissues. Analytical Biochemistry. 2010;**400**(1):110-117. DOI: 10.1016/j.ab.2010.01.014

[112] Pikor LA, Enfield KSS, Cameron H, Lam WL. DNA extraction from paraffin embedded material for genetic and epigenetic analyses. Journal of Visualized Experiments. 2011;**49**: 2763. DOI: 10.3791/2763

[113] Patel PG, Selvarajah S, Boursalie S, et al. Preparation of formalin-fixed paraffin-embedded tissue cores for both RNA and DNA extraction. Journal of Visualized Experiments. 2016;**114**:54299. DOI: 10.3791/54299

[114] Tomonari K, Sonoda A, Ikehara A, et al. Comparison of methods for the extraction of DNA from formalin-fixed paraffin-embedded tissues for human identification. Japanese Journal of Forensic Science and Technology. 2017. Article ID: 734. DOI: http://doi.org/10.3408/jafst.734

[115] Cecchetto G, Bajanowski T, Cecchi R, et al. Back to the future – Part 1. The medico-legal autopsy from ancient civilization to the post-genomic era. International Journal of Legal Medicine. 2017;**131**(4):1069-1083. DOI: 10.1007/s00414-017-1584-8

[116] Ferrara SD, Cecchetto G, Cecchi R, et al. Back to the future – Part 2. Post-mortem assessment and evolutionary role of the bio-medicolegal sciences. International Journal of Legal Medicine. 2017;**131**(4):1085-1101. DOI: 10.1007/s00414-017-1585-7

[117] Pickrahn I. Kreindl G, Müller E, et al. Contamination when collecting trace evidence – An issue more relevant than ever? Forensic Science International: Genetics Supplement Series. 2015;**5**:e603-e604. DOI: https://doi.org/10.1016/j.fsigss.2015.09.238

[118] Helmus J, Bajanowski T, Poetsch M. DNA transfer – A never ending story. A study on scenarios involving a second person as carrier. International Journal of Legal Medicine. 2016;**130**(1):121-125. DOI: 10.1007/s00414-015-1284-1, https://doi.org/10.1007/s00414-015-1284-1

[119] Benschop CC, Haned H, Yoo SY, Sijen T. Evaluation of samples comprising minute amounts of DNA. Science & Justice. 2015;**55**(5):316-322. DOI: 10.1016/j.scijus.2015.05.002

[120] Hansson O, Gill P. Characterisation of artefacts and drop-in events using STR-validator and single-cell analysis. Forensic Science International. Genetics. 2017;**30**:57-65. DOI: 10.1016/j.fsigen.2017.04.015. (Epub Apr 21, 2017)

Chapter 9

Application of CO-oximeter for Forensic Samples

Hiroshi Kinoshita, Naoko Tanaka, Ayaka Takakura, Mostofa Jamal, Asuka Ito, Mitsuru Kumihashi, Shoji Kimura, Kunihiko Tsutsui, Shuji Matsubara and Kiyoshi Ameno

Additional information is available at the end of the chapter

http://dx.doi.org/10.5772/intechopen.71182

Abstract

CO-oximeter is routinely used in clinical practice, and it has been applied in the field of forensic medicine. It is a simultaneous and nondestructive technique for the analysis of total hemoglobin (Hb) and various Hb species, such as oxyhemoglobin, reduced hemoglobin, carboxyhemoglobin, and methemoglobin. It automatically measures the proportion of each species of Hb and oxygen contents. This is an easy, rapid, and convenient way as the laboratory test. Since there are many advantages such as no necessity of sample preparation, easy handling, and portability, it may provide valuable information for forensic diagnosis. In the present paper, we discuss about the diagnostic application of CO-oximeter in the field of forensic medicine.

Keywords: CO-oximeter, forensic diagnosis, carbon monoxide poisoning, hypothermia, methemoglobin

1. Introduction

CO-oximeter is widely used in clinical practice [1–5]. It would be measurable total hemoglobin (Hb) and various Hb species, such as oxyhemoglobin (O_2Hb), reduced hemoglobin (HHb), carboxyhemoglobin (COHb), and methemoglobin (MetHb), simultaneously. This is an easy, rapid, and convenient way as the laboratory test, and it provides valuable information for clinical diagnosis. It is widely used in clinical laboratory, emergency department, intensive care unit, or cardiac catheterization laboratory for the evaluation of general status including the ability of oxygenation or ventilation [1–5].

It has been reported that CO-oximeter is applied in a field of forensic diagnosis [6–30]. In the present chapter, we discuss about the diagnostic application of CO-oximeter in the field of forensic medicine.

2. Principle of the CO-oximeter

The CO-oximeter is a spectrophotometer that determines hemoglobin derivatives in blood by measuring absorbance at selected wavelength [1, 2, 31, 32]. The Hb solutions obey the Lambert-Beer Law, and the absorbance measured at selected wavelength is the sum of the absorbance of each Hb derivative [31–36]. The wavelength is selected by the combination of absorption maxima and isosbestic points [37]. The concentration of four Hb derivatives (O_2Hb, HHb, COHb, and MetHb) is determined by measuring absorbance at four wavelengths [33].

The CO-oximeter is included in the routine toxicological examination in daily forensic practice, as it is not necessary for the sample pretreatment or any reagent.

3. Forensic application of CO-oximeter

Since the O_2Hb in the postmortem heart blood was usually very low (under 10%) in most of the cases, postmortem blood gas analysis is less valuable for interpretation of cause of death [13]. However, the composition of Hb provides valuable information for forensic diagnosis.

We have been using the AVOX4000 (AVOX; International Technidyne Corporation, NJ, USA), which monitors seven wavelengths (488.4, 520.1, 562.4, 585.2, 597.5, 621.7, and 671.7 nm) in the visible region for the determination of various Hb species [24]. This portable CO-oximeter (**Figure 1**) requires 50 μl of blood for single measurement, and it may be a valid option in case of difficult blood sampling due to severe blood loss. Since there are many advantages such as no necessity of sample preparation, easy handling, and portability, it is suitable for forensic practice. It automatically analyzes the proportion of each species of Hb and oxygen contents.

3.1. Carbon monoxide (CO) poisoning

CO is an odorless, colorless and nonirritable gas, mainly produced by incomplete combustion of fuels or carbon compounds [38, 39]. CO is second most common cause of death among non-medical poisonings in United States [40], and the leading cause of poisoning death in Japan [41, 42]. It includes accidental or suicidal poisoning, and the postmortem investigation for CO poisoning and its related death are important for forensic practice.

CO binds to hemoglobin and forms COHb (represented as a percentage of the total Hb) following inhalation of CO gas [39, 43, 44]. As the affinity of CO for Hb is 200–300 times greater than that for oxygen, the toxicity of CO is mainly thought to be the decrease the capacity of oxygen transport, and it causes impairment of oxygen supply in tissue level [39, 43–46]. In a recent study, it may be involved interference with ferroproteins such as myoglobin and cytochrome oxidases [43, 45, 46].

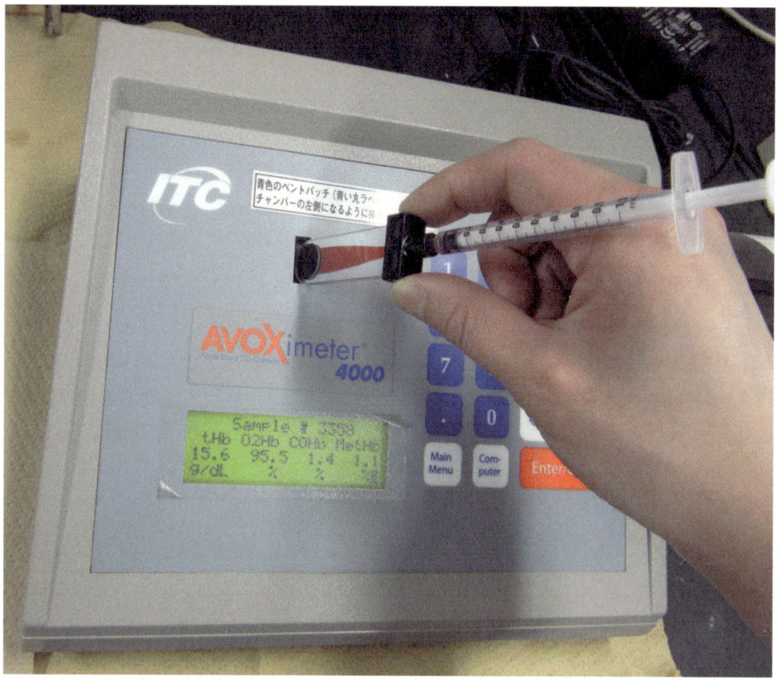

Figure 1. Portable oximeter (AVOX 4000).

CO-Hb (%)	Clinical symptoms
<1-2	Normal range (due to endogenous production)
<10	Smoker's blood (no symptom)
10–20	Headache
20–40	Headache, nausea, vomiting
40-	Severe symptoms
50–60	Coma, convulsions
60-	Cardiorespiratory depression or failure, often fatal

Table 1. Level of carboxyhemoglobin (COHb) and symptoms.

Table 1 shows the relationship between toxic symptoms and COHb levels [39, 46]. However, it is not an absolute reference value, and large individual difference was observed in fatal level. Severe symptoms such as convulsion, deep coma, and cardiovascular failure are observed around 50% of COHb level. The fatal COHb levels are more than 50–60%, and its values are important for the diagnosis of fatal CO poisoning [46]. However, lethal level has large variation. Elderly people may die at relatively low concentration in some cases [46]. It may be involved to pathological status such as anemia, coronary artery disease, and respiratory insufficiency [46]. Autopsy findings indicate that blood, organs, and muscle will be cherry red color, as a result of COHb formation. Other findings such as pulmonary edema and generalized organ congestion are also observed [46].

The application of oximeter in fatal CO poisoning case has been reported [6, 7, 10–13, 15–20, 22–29]. Various methods such as spectrophotometric method and gas chromatography have been also employed for the identification and quantification of CO [43, 47]. There was a good correlation between the COHb values obtained by AVOX and by the conventional method [23]. No arterial-venous difference of COHb concentration was observed at the level less than 75% of COHb [23] and in animal experiments [48].

In a forensic practice, we sometimes treat various kinds of denatured blood samples such as from the putrefied bodies or thermo-coagulated one. As the COHb is relatively stable under the storage in cool and dark conditions, it would be accurately measurable less than 2 years under the storage in fridges [22, 49], and it is possible for rough estimation of COHb levels in thermo-coagulated blood with CO oximeter [6, 12]. In recent study, it has been reported that splenic blood, which is obtained by manual squeezing, is applicable for alternative matrix for COHb measurement using AVOX [29].

3.2. Fire-related cases

The victims by fire will die not only from the thermal injury but also from inhalation of the toxic substances such as CO, cyanide, nitric oxide, phosgene, and others and reduction of the atmospheric oxygen [46]. When the organic material burn but access of oxygen is limited in fire, large amount of CO is produced by the incomplete combustion. The COHb level in fire-related cases is an important aspect [46]. The presence of CO in circulating blood and carbon particle in the air passages indicates that the victim was alive after the fire began [46]. It is a valuable indicator in fire-related cases. The COHb levels in blood of the fire victim depend on various factors such as CO concentration in atmosphere, time of exposure, and oxygen contents [46].

It has been reported that marked arteriovenous and centroperipheral difference of COHb were observed in the group of above ca.70% of COHb [11]. It seems to be that inhalation of CO-rich air immediately causes acute heart failure [11]. On the other hand, COHb levels in victim were lower in flash fires or open-air petrol involved cases. The quick measurement of COHb using CO-oximeter in victim of fire-related case provides valuable information for forensic diagnosis.

3.3. Hypothermia

There is little or no diagnostic findings in cases of fatal hypothermic death [14, 28, 30, 46, 50–55]. It has been reported that the blood in left cardiac chamber is bright red compared to that in right cardiac chamber [28, 30, 50, 51, 53, 56]. This color difference between left and right heart blood is a common characteristic sign of hypothermic death. This finding was observed in approximately 95% of hypothermic death cases [30, 50, 53]. This color difference is formed by many factors such as decrease of body temperature, binding of oxygen to Hb, and inhalation of cold air before death [30, 50]. The blood in left heart has usually higher oxygen contents than that in right heart. The lower body temperature keeps the antemortem composition of Hb following death, and it also enhances the oxygen binding to Hb [30, 50, 53].

The O_2Hb saturation level could increase as a result of cardiopulmonary resuscitation or administration of oxygen. We have to exclude the following cases such as subjected to body rewarming, long postmortem interval, and received cardiopulmonary resuscitation, for forensic diagnostic application of CO-oximeter [30].

It has been proposed that the diagnostic criterion of hypothermic death, designating O_2Hb in left cardiac blood ≥36% as a basic condition, with the difference in the O_2Hb saturation level between left and right heart blood ≥13% or O_2Hb saturation ratio between left and right heart blood ≥1.8, as a complementary condition [30]. This finding reflects the final balance of oxygen uptake and consumption in the dying process, and the pathophysiological status of the victim would be obtained by the application of CO-oximeter for forensic diagnosis.

3.4. Evaluation of MetHb

MetHb is a form of Hb in which ferric iron (Fe^{3+}) is carried in its heme group [57]. It is formed by the exposure to oxidizing agents such as nitrates, nitrites, or chlorates [57–59]. MetHb may also arise from genetic, dietary, or idiopathic etiologies [57–59]. It causes impairment of O_2 and CO_2 transport, leading to tissue or cellular hypoxia [57–59]. High levels of MetHb have been observed in cases of fire and poisoning by various oxidizing agents such as vehicle exhaust (containing nitric oxide and nitrogen dioxide), nitrate, and chlorate [60–64]. We should also take into consideration about the stability of MetHb. The formation of MetHb by postmortem oxidation of heme-protein has been reported [8]. On the other hand, high COHb containing blood is considered to have heat resistant properties, and the formation of MetHb is lower [65]. Spontaneous reduction of MetHb in blood sample due to the enzyme activity has also been reported [66]. We have to consider them for the interpretation of the MetHb value.

Measurement of MetHb using the conventional spectrophotometric method [67] is relatively complicated procedure. On the other hand, CO-oximeter is routinely used in clinical practice [2, 3, 5] and has also been applied in forensic practice [8, 64]. **Table 2** shows

MetHb (%)	Clinical symptom
<1–2	Normal range (no symptom)
10–15	Cyanosis
20-	Headache, dyspnea, tachycardia, tachypnea
40–50	Mental derangement, metabolic acidosis
50-	Coma, convulsion
70-	Death

Table 2. Level of methemoglobin (MetHb) and symptoms.

the relationship between toxic symptoms and MetHb concentration [57–59, 68]. The blood MetHb concentration is less than 1–2% in normal healthy subjects, and fatal concentration of MetHb in blood has been reported higher than 70% [57–59, 68]. Blood MetHb concentration provides useful toxicological information for forensic diagnosis. From these results, additional toxicological examination for oxidizing agent may be requested to the forensic toxicologist.

4. Conclusion and future perspective

We have discussed about the application of CO-oximeter in forensic practice. The postmortem oximetric profiles may be considered to reflect the final balance of oxygen uptake and consumption in the dying process [13]. Those data may be valuable for interpretation in some cause of death and provides valuable information for forensic diagnosis. Further applications in the fields of forensic practice can be expected.

Acknowledgements

This work was supported by JSPS KAKENHI Grant-in-Aid for Scientific Research (C) Number 15 K08873.

Conflict of interest

The authors declare that there is no conflict of interest regarding the publication of this paper.

Author details

Hiroshi Kinoshita[1*], Naoko Tanaka[1], Ayaka Takakura[1], Mostofa Jamal[1], Asuka Ito[1], Mitsuru Kumihashi[1], Shoji Kimura[1], Kunihiko Tsutsui[2], Shuji Matsubara[3] and Kiyoshi Ameno[1]

*Address all correspondence to: kinochin@med.kagawa-u.ac.jp

1 Department of Forensic Medicine, Faculty of Medicine, Kagawa University, Miki, Kagawa, Japan

2 Health Sciences, Faculty of Medicine, Kagawa University, Miki, Kagawa, Japan

3 Community Health Care Education Support Center, and Postgraduate Clinical Education Center, Kagawa University Hospital, Miki, Kagawa, Japan

References

[1] Zijlstra WG, Buursma A, Zwart A. Performance of an automated six-wavelength photometer (Radiometer OSM3) for routine measurement of hemoglobin derivatives. Clinical Chemistry. 1988;**34**:149-152

[2] Mahoney JJ, Vreman HJ, Stevenson DK, Van Kessel AL. Measurement of carboxyhemoglobin and total hemoglobin by five specialized spectrophotometers (CO-oximeters) in comparison with reference methods. Clinical Chemistry. 1993;**39**:1693-1700

[3] Gong AK. Near-patient measurements of methemoglobin, oxygen saturation, and total hemoglobin: Evaluation of a new instrument for adult and neonatal intensive care. Critical Care Medicine. 1995;**23**:190-201

[4] Touger M, Gallagher EJ, Tyrell J. Relationship between venous and arterial carboxyhemoglobin levels in patients with suspected carbon monoxide poisoning. Annals of Emergency Medicine. 1995;**25**:481-483

[5] Bailey SR, Russell RN, Martinez A. Evaluation of the avoximeter: Precision, long-term stability, and use without heparin. Journal of Clinical Monitoring. 1997;**13**:191-198

[6] Freireich AW, Landau D. Carbon monoxide determination in postmortem clotted blood. Journal of Forensic Sciences. 1971;**16**:112-119

[7] Okada M, Okada T, Ide K. Utilization of a CO-oximeter in the medico-legal field. Nihon Houigaku Zasshi. 1985;**39**:318-325

[8] Okada M, Okada T, Kawaguchi N, Ide K. Studies of methemoglobin production in the blood of dead burn victims. Nihon Houigaku Zasshi. 1986;**40**:124-128

[9] Ohshima T, Takayasu T, Nishigami J, Lin Z, Kondo T, Nagano T. Application of hemoglobin analysis by CO-oximeter to medico-legal practice with special reference to diagnosis of asphyxia. Nihon Houigaku Zasshi. 1992;**46**:382-388

[10] Higuchi T, Noguchi K, Maeda H. An evaluation of analyzed data of hemoglobin derivatives by CO-oximeter in medico-legal autopsy. Nihon Houigaku Zasshi. 1992;**46**:416-418

[11] Maeda H, Fukita K, Oritani S, Nagai K, Zhu BL. An evaluation of post-mortem oxymetry in fire victims. Forensic Science International. 1996;**81**:201-209

[12] Oritani S, Nagai K, Zhu BL, Maeda H. Estimation of carboxyhemoglobin concentrations in thermo-coagulated blood on a CO-oximeter system: an experimental study. Forensic Science International. 1996;**83**:211-218

[13] Maeda H, Fukita K, Oritani S, Ishida K, Zhu BL. Evaluation of post-mortem oxymetry with reference to the causes of death. Forensic Science International. 1997;**87**:201-210

[14] Shimizu K, Mizukami H, Fukushima T, Sasaki M, Shiono H. Use of a CO-oximeter for forensic diagnosis of hypothermia. Nihon Houigaku Zasshi. 1998;**52**:196-201

[15] Lee CW, Tam JCN, Kung LK, Yim LK. Validity of CO-oximetric determination of carboxy-haemoglobin in putrefying blood and body cavity fluid. Forensic Science International. 2003;**132**:153-156

[16] Brehmer C, Iten PX. Rapid determination of carboxyhemoglobin in blood by Oximeter. Forensic Science International. 2003;**133**:179-181

[17] Watanabe N, Terazawa K, Sakaihara M. Blood storage for forensic hemoglobin analysis using CO-oximeter. Hokkaido Igaku Zasshi. 2003;**78**:289-295

[18] Watanabe N. Medico-legal application of hemoglobin analysis using CO-oximeter. Hokkaido Igaku Zasshi. 2003;**78**:557-566

[19] Olson KN, Hillyer MA, Kloss JS, Geiselhart RJ, Apple FS. Accident or arson: Is Co-oximetry reliable for carboxyhemoglobin measurement postmortem? Clinical Chemistry. 2010;**56**: 515-520

[20] Tanaka N, Ameno K, Jamal M, Ohkubo E, Kumihashi M, Kinoshita H. Application of oximeter AVOX 4000 for the determination of CO-Hb in the forensic practice. The Research and Practice in Forensic Medicine. 2010;**53**:39-43

[21] Tanaka N, Ameno K, Jamal M, Kumihashi M, Kinoshita H. Application of oximeter AVOX 4000 in the forensic practice (report 2): Diagnosis for hypothermia. The Research and Practice in Forensic Medicine. 2011;**54**:205-209

[22] Tanaka N, Ameno K, Jamal M, Kumihashi M, Miyatake N, Kinoshita H. Effects of sampling methods and storage on the value of oxyhemoglobin ratio and carboxyhemoglobin ratio. The Research and Practice in Forensic Medicine. 2012;**55**:51-55

[23] Kinoshita H, Tanaka N, Jamal M, Kumihashi M, Ameno K. Evaluation of carboxyhemoglobin (CO-Hb) by oximeter in forensic practice. In: DiLoreto D, Corcoran I, editors. Carbon Monoxide Source, Uses and Hazards. New York: Nova Science Publishers, Inc.; 2012. p. 109-116

[24] Fujihara J, Kinoshita H, Tanaka N, Yasuda T, Takeshita H. Accuracy and usefulness of the AVOXimeter 4000 as routine analysis of carboxyhemoglobin. Journal of Forensic Sciences. 2013;**58**:1047-1049

[25] Fujihara J, Hasegawa M, Kato T, Miura M, Iida K, Kinoshita H, Tanaka N, Takeshita H. A case of drowning lacking typical autopsy findings of carbon monoxide poisoning despite the high CO concentration. Forensic Toxicology. 2013;**31**:180-182

[26] Nakagawa H, Maebashi K, Fukui K, Ochiai E, Iwadate K. Applicability of a new CO oximeter to forensic autopsy cases. Acta Criminologicae et Medicinae Legalis Japonica. 2013;**79**:16-21

[27] Tanaka N, Ameno K, Jamal M, Kumihashi M, Miyatake N, Kinoshita H. Effects of sample dilution on the value of carboxyhemoglobin ratio. Japanese Journal of Forensic Pathology. 2014;**20**:39-40

[28] Kanoto-Nishimaki Y, Saito H, Watanabe-Aoyagi M, Toda R, Iwadate K. Investigation of oxyhemoglobin and carboxyhemoglobin ratios in right and left cardiac blood for diagnosis of fatal hypothermia and death by fire. Legal Medicine (Tokyo). 2014;**16**:321-325

[29] Tanaka N, Kinoshita H, Jamal M, Takakura A, Kumihashi M, Miyatake N, Ameno K. Squeezed splenic blood sampling as an alternative method for carboxyhemoglobin measurement. Romanian Journal of Legal Medicine. 2015;**23**:106-108

[30] Yajima D, Asari M, Okuda K, Maseda C, Yamada H, Ichimaru C, Matsubara K, Shiono H, Iwase H, Makino Y, Shimizu K. An objective approach using three indexes for determining fatal hypothermia due to cold exposure; statistical analysis of oxyhemoglobin saturation data. Legal Medicine (Tokyo). 2015;**17**:451-458

[31] Yukawa N, Suzuoka T, Saito T, Forrest ARW, Osawa M, Takeichi S. Data processing in CO-oximeters that use overdetermined systems. Clinical Chemistry. 1997;**43**:189-190

[32] Yukawa N, Suzuoka T, Saito T, Forrest ARW, Osawa M, Takeichi S. Current CO-oximeter. Forensic Science International. 1998;**94**:211-215

[33] Brown LJ. A new instrument for the simultaneous measurement of total hemoglobin, % oxyhemoglobin, % carboxyhemoglobin, % methemoglobin, and oxygen content in whole blood. IEEE Transactions on Biomedical Engineering. 1980;**27**:132-138

[34] Zwart A, Buursma A, van Kampen EJ, Oeseburg B, van der Ploeg PHW, Zijlstra WG. A multi-wavelength spectrophotometric method for the simultaneous determination of five haemoglobin derivatives. Journal of Clinical Chemistry and Clinical Biochemistry. 1981;**319**:457-463

[35] Zwart A, Buursma A, van EJ, Zijlstra WG. Multicomponent analysis of hemoglobin derivatives with reversed-optics spectrophotometer. Clinical Chemistry. 1984;**30**:373-379

[36] Zwart A, van Kampen EJ, Zijilstra WG. Results of routine determination of clinically significant hemoglobin derivatives by multicomponent analysis. Clinical Chemistry. 1986;**32**:972-978

[37] Brunelle JA, Moran RF. A manufacturer replies. Clinical Chemistry. 1997;**43**:190-191

[38] Baselt RC. Disposition of Toxic Drugs and Chemicals in Man. 8th ed. Foster City: Biochemical Publications; 2008

[39] Elenhorn MJ, Barceloux DG. Medical Toxicology Diagnosis and Treatment of Human Poisoning. New York: Elsevier; 1988

[40] Sircar K, Clower J, Shin MK, Bailey C, King M, Yip F. Carbon monoxide poisoning deaths in the United States, 1999 to 2012. The American Journal of Emergency Medicine. 2015;**33**:1140-1145

[41] Ministry of Health, Labour and Walfare. Vital Statistics of Japan. Tokyo: Health, Labour and Walfare Statistics Association; 1998-2015.

[42] Ito T, Nakamura Y. Death from carbon monoxide poisoning in Japan between 1968-2007 through data from vital statistics. Journal of Japanese Society for Emergency Medicine. 2010;**13**:275-282

[43] World Health Organization. Environmental Health Criteria 213, Carbon Monoxide. 2nd ed. Geneva: World Health Organization; 1999

[44] Powers RH, Dean DE. Forensic Toxicology Mechanism and Pathology. Boca Raton: CRC Press; 2016

[45] Tomaszewski C. Carbon monoxide. In: Nelson LS et al., editors. Goldfrank's Toxicologic Emergencies. 9th ed. New York, Chicago: McGraw-Hill; 2011. p. 1658-1670

[46] Saukko P, Knight B. Knight's Forensic Pathology. 4th ed. Boca Raton, FL: CRC Press; 2016

[47] Akane A, Fukui Y. A review on the development of carboxyhemoglobin analysis. The Research and Practice in Forensic Medicine. 1985;**28**:185-190

[48] Lopetz DM, Weingarten-Arams JS, Singer LP, Conway EE. Relationship between arterial, mixed venous, and internal jugular carboxyhemoglobin concentrations at low, medium, and high concentrations in a piglet model of carbon monoxide toxicity. Critical Care Medicine. 2000;**28**:1998-2001

[49] Kunsman GW, Presses CL, Prodriguez P. Carbon monoxide stability in stored postmortem blood samples. Journal of Analytical Toxicology. 2000;**24**:572-578

[50] Shimizu K, Shiono H, Fukushima T, Sasaki M. Diagnosis of fatal hypothermia—Differences in color between blood from the right and left ventricles and prevalence of Wischnewski's Spot. Acta Criminologicae et Medicinae Legalis Japonica. 1996;**62**:157-160

[51] Mizukami H, Shimizu K, Shiono H, Uezono T, Sasaki M. Forensic diagnosis of death from cold. Legal Medicine (Tokyo). 1999;**1**:204-209

[52] Türk EE, Sperhake JP, Pueschel K, Tsokos M. An approach to the evaluation of fatal hypothermia. Forensic Science, Medicine, and Pathology. 2005;**1**:31-35

[53] Shiono H, Shimizu K. Necropsy and autopsy diagnosis of fatal hypothermia. The Research and Practice in Forensic Medicine. 2007;**50**:1-7

[54] Funayama M. Diagnosis of hypothermia. Nihon Hōigaku Zasshi. 2008;**62**:145-154

[55] Turk EE. Hypothermia. Forensic Science, Medicine, and Pathology. 2010;**6**:106-115

[56] Iwadate K. Death from cold. In: Nagao M et al., editors. New Essentials of Forensic Medicine. 5th ed. Tokyo: Ishiyaku Publishers Inc; 2012. p. 189-192

[57] Wright RO, Lewander WJ, Woolf AD. Methemoglobinemia: etiology, pharmacology, and clinical management. Annals of Emergency Medicine. 1999;**34**:646-656

[58] Blanc PD. Methemoglobinemia. In: Olson KR, editor. Poisoning & Drug Overdose. 5th ed. New York: Lange Medical Books/McGraw-Hill; 2007. p. 262-264

[59] Price DP. Methemoglobin inducers. In: Nelson LS et al., editors. Goldfrank's Toxicologic Emergencies. 9th ed. New York, Chicago: McGraw-Hill; 2011. p. 1698-1707

[60] Saito T, Takeichi S, Osawa M, Yukawa N, Huang X-L. A case of fatal methemoglobinemia of unknown origin but presumably due to ingestion of nitrate. International Journal of Legal Medicine. 2000;**113**:164-167

[61] Suyama H, Morikawa S, Noma-Tanaka S, Adachi H, Kawano Y, Kaneko K, Ishihara S. Methemglobinemia induced by automobile exhaust fumes. Journal of Anesthesia. 2005;**19**:333-335

[62] Vevelstad M, Morild I. Lethal methemoglobinemia and automobile exhaust inhalation. Forensic Science International. 2009;**187**:e1-e5

[63] Kinoshita H, Yoshioka N, Kuse A, Nishiguchi M, Tanaka N, Jamal M, Kumihashi M, Nagasaki Y, Ueno Y, Ameno K. A fatal case of severe methemoglobinemia presumably due to chlorate ingestion. Soudní Lékarství. 2011;**56**:43-44

[64] Nishiguchi M, Nushida H, Okudaira N, Nishio H. An autopsy case of fatal methemoglobinemia due to ingestion of sodium nitrite. Journal of Forensic Research. 2015;**6**:262

[65] Shigezane J. Effects of heating on methemoglobin contents in blood. Nihon Houigaku Zasshi. 1985;**39**:1-5

[66] Fukui Y, Yamamoto Y, Mastubara K. Reduction with lapse of time of methemoglobin in blood sample. Nihon Houigaku Zasshi. 1980;**34**:563-568

[67] Sato K. A method for determination of methemoglobin in blood containing carboxyhemoglobin. Nihon Houigaku Zasshi. 1983;**37**:133-144

[68] Sato K. Methemoglobin. In: Suzuki O, Watanabe K, editors. Drugs and Poisons in Humans, A Handbook of Practical Analysis. Berlin, Heidelberg: Springer-Verlag; 2002. p. 655-657